Safe and Effective Staffing Levels for the Allied Health Professions

A PRACTICAL GUIDE

ROBERT JONES
PhD, MPhil, BA, FCSP, Grad.Dip.Phys, CHSM

FIONA JENKINS
MA, FCSP, NEBS(M), CHSM, Grad.Dip.Phys

Otmoor Publishing
Oxford

Otmoor Publishing Ltd
Oxford OX5 2RD
United Kingdom

© 2014 Robert Jones and Fiona Jenkins

Robert Jones and Fiona Jenkins have asserted their right under the Copyright, Designs and Patents Act 1988 to be identified as the authors of this work.

All rights reserved. No part of this publication may be reproduced, stored in a retrieval system or transmitted, in any form or by any means, electronic, mechanical, photocopying, recording or otherwise, without the prior permission of the copyright owner.

British Library Cataloguing Publication Data

A catalogue record for this book is available from the British Library.

ISBN-13 978 1 910303 00 9

Typeset and designed by Darkriver Design, Auckland, New Zealand
Printed by Printondemand-Worldwide.com

Contents

List of Figures and Tables	vi
Foreword	vii
Preface	ix
About the Authors	xi
Books in the Allied Health Professions Essential Guides *Series by Robert Jones and Fiona Jenkins*	xii
Abbreviations	xiii

1 Introduction — 1
Introduction — 1
About this book — 2
Origins of our approach — 3
Conclusion — 6

2 Key Investigations and Reports — 7
The Francis Report — 7
The Berwick Report — 8
The Keogh Report — 8
The Cavendish Review — 9
Wales, Scotland and Northern Ireland — 9
Other comment and conclusion — 11

3 Media Focus and Reporting — 13

4 Where do the Professions Stand? Statements, Publications and Recommendations — 17
Nursing — 17
Medical services — 22
Allied health professions — 23
An international perspective — 27

5 Are there Staffing Level Methodologies for the AHPs? — 33
A case study — 33

6 Methodology for Determining Safe and Effective Staffing Levels for the AHPs – The Jones/Jenkins Approach — 43

- Introduction — 43
  - What it's not — 44
  - What is our main aim? — 44
  - The four countries of the UK — 44
- Basis of our methodology, the concept – what you do — 44
  - The steps for calculation — 45
- The AHP working week in the UK — 46
- Workload data examples — 47
  - Example 1 – A typical AHP — 47
  - Example 2 – A service department with 10 WTE — 47
  - Example 3 – A worked capacity example — 48
  - Example 4 – an example from NZ — 48
  - Example 5 – an NZ Service with 10 WTE — 48
- Staff activity analysis — 50
  - Tips for implementation — 52
  - AHP services activity sample pro forma: briefing notes — 52
  - The Form Part 1 – General information — 52
  - The Form Part 2 – Patient-related activity — 53
  - The Form Part 3 – Non-patient-related activity — 53
  - The Form Part 4 – About your contracted hours and caseload — 55
  - Example of reports from activity sample data — 55
  - Data and information management — 55
  - Application of activity sampling in the context of staffing level determination — 56
  - Average levels of patient-related activity — 56
- Benchmarking AHP services — 56
  - Introducing our Benchmarking Tool — 57
  - How to use the tool – briefing notes — 57
- The 7-days-a-week question – what staffing level? — 68
  - Care pathways in the context of staffing level determination — 69
- Business cases — 69
- Conclusion — 70

Appendix 1 HCPC professions — 71

Appendix 2 Principles for computerised information systems for AHP services — 72

Appendix 3 Key elements in a business case — 76
  Elements in a business case – an example — 76

Appendix 4 Suggested data checklist for AHP managers and leaders   79

Appendix 5 Numbers of Hospital Beds and Staff per 1000 population
– examples of calculation   81

References   83
Index   89

List of Figures and Tables

Figures

1	AHP services activity sample pro forma	51
2	Subdivision of staff time by staff band	54
3	Subdivision of staff time; all staff	54
4	Comparison of out-patient staff: patient-related to non-patient-related activity by Band 7 and Band 5, physiotherapy out-patient service	55
5	Five to seven day workforce redeployment	68

Tables

1	Your Organisation	59
2	Professional group and staffing	61
3	In-patient services	63
4	Out-patient services	65
5	Community services	67

Foreword

I am delighted to welcome this very timely and significant book by Robert and Fiona – two nationally and internationally respected and highly experienced allied health professionals (AHPs) with great expertise – which will assist both United Kingdom (UK) and international AHP managers and leaders and others in one of the biggest health challenges of today … what are the safe and effective staffing levels which will ensure the provision of quality AHP services? And what are the credible methodologies for determining staffing levels given the huge variations that exist in different health settings and between different organisations?

I have been involved in the challenges of workforce planning and staffing levels for AHPs and nursing for over 35 years, most recently during more than 15 years as the former Chief Executive Officer of the UK's Chartered Society of Physiotherapy, with its 52,000 members. Yet determining staffing levels is neither simple nor obvious, nor is there any standard, nationally or internationally agreed methodology in nursing, medicine or AHPs. If it was that simple, methods would have been agreed years ago. The reality is that the provision of health services differs significantly depending on the hospital or community setting; patient need and level of dependency; patient population, size and turnover; age profile; types of specialties; skill mix; and, crucially, the levels of healthcare funding available.

What makes the whole agenda – and therefore this book – so urgent for AHP managers and leaders in the UK is the recent health scandals centred around inadequate and unsafe nursing staff numbers for care of the rapidly growing numbers of frail older people needing care in hospitals. This has resulted in several hard hitting reports during 2013, including the major Francis Report, plus the Berwick, Cavendish and Keogh Reports. Similar pressures also exist internationally.

The result has been the search for possible statutory minimum staffing levels – which are unlikely to work – or the urgent commission of UK research to agree a new, credible and sophisticated nurse staffing methodology. This could take years to produce.

The other important context worldwide has been the rapid growth in the demand for health services from the population, including older people, during a period of deep economic recession where the UK and other governments are either cutting healthcare funding or, at best, keeping them static while demand escalates.

For the AHPs the challenge is twofold. Firstly, since the national spotlight is on safe and effective nursing numbers, AHP managers and leaders need to be able to challenge firmly any local attempts to improve nursing safety by reductions in AHP staff numbers, making these services unsafe and ineffective. Secondly, AHP managers and leaders need to be equipped with the practical processes and a credible methodology to determine the appropriate safe and effective staffing levels for providing a quality service for patients locally with all its variations. AHP services have a major part to play in keeping people out of hospital, maintaining their independence or rehabilitating them after injury or illness.

Robert and Fiona's book is a major step forward for the AHPs in dealing with the immediate challenges they face on staffing levels. It will equip managers and leaders of AHPs and other healthcare disciplines with the means to produce a well argued and credible set of proposals for senior healthcare management. Further national research over the next few years may possibly produce further methodologies, but today, this book is a very welcome and important addition to the literature which fills a gap for all AHP managers and leaders both nationally and internationally.

Phil Gray FCSP (Hon), MSc, BSc

Preface

Patient safety, ensuring sufficient time for consistently good quality effective care and care provided with compassion and respect for patients' dignity, must be at the heart of all healthcare and be central to the allied health professional's work.

The Francis Report on serious failings at the Mid Staffordshire NHS Foundation Trust and subsequent reports including the Berwick Report and the Keogh Report (all published during 2013) drew attention to the correlation between patient safety and staffing levels on hospital wards, highlighting the need to ensure patient safety is of paramount concern for healthcare providers, planners and commissioners. This has raised awareness, not only of policy makers and the media, but also of the general public about standards of care in hospitals, bringing a much more critical analysis of service providers and expectations about the quality of care that should be provided. This national emphasis on quality of care and staffing levels has also come to the fore at a time when healthcare services face significant financial challenges and pressures.

Although the nursing profession was largely under the spotlight, allied health professions (AHPs) are also key providers of health and social care and it is important that they be treated as an integral part of the care provision picture, and consequently staffing levels determination.

To date, there has been no nationally or internationally accepted consistent methodology adopted to determine AHPs staffing levels, giving rise to much variance between different providers and services.

For many years we have been working on the development of a – what we believe to be – robust, evidence-based and logical approach to resolve this complex issue, including the development of several tried and tested tools which can be used in staffing levels, workforce determination and in a wide range of other AHP management and leadership practice.

The National Institute for Health and Care Excellence (NICE) has been asked to review any available evidence and to produce definitive guidance on safe and effective/efficient staffing levels in a range of healthcare settings during 2014. We hope that our approach described in this book will support AHP managers and leaders, commissioners and service planners, and all those working in workforce determination in all sectors of healthcare provision. We also believe that the methodology and the concepts on which it is based will provide a useful tool for NICE and a wide range of other policy makers working on workforce development. The methodology is applicable to all healthcare settings where AHPs are providing services, and is equally applicable to AHP services throughout the UK. When we were undertaking the scoping work of published literature, possible methodologies, policies, statements and processes for this book, we scoped both nationally and internationally and there was a great deal of interest from overseas in the work we were undertaking. We hope, therefore, that our approach might also be of interest and use to our AHP colleagues in many situations around the world.

We are pleased that, given the recognition of the importance of staffing level determination to good quality, safe, effective, compassionate, caring services, the time has come for us to publish our work in this area. We hope that our methodology and the concepts which underpin it will help many AHPs and others wrestling with this complex and difficult work.

We wholeheartedly thank Gillian Nineham, Otmoor Publishing Ltd for guidance through the publication process, for her great expertise, encouragement and help in bringing the book to fruition.

Robert Jones and Fiona Jenkins
May 2014

About the Authors

Dr Robert Jones PhD, MPhil, BA, FCSP, Grad.Dip.Phys, CHSM
Governor, Moorfields Eye Hospital NHS Foundation Trust.
Director, JJ Consulting Healthcare Management Ltd.
Recent former Head of Therapy Services Directorate, East Sussex Healthcare NHS Trust.
Robert is a healthcare management and leadership consultant with over 40 years' experience as a physiotherapist, including 30 years' senior management and leadership experience. Robert was a Council member, Vice-Chair and Chairman of the Chartered Society of Physiotherapy and Vice-President. He was the first Registrant physiotherapy member of the Health Professions Council and was seconded to the Commission for Health Improvement as AHP Consultant/advisor. He has represented Allied Health on a Department of Health Information Authority Project Board and several other Department of Health groups. Robert has published widely on management/leadership, clinical topics, and IM&T including peer reviewed articles. He is an Honorary Fellow of the University of Brighton and Plymouth University.

Fiona Jenkins MA (Dist), FCSP, NEBS(M), CHSM, Grad.Dip.Phys
Fiona is Executive Director of Therapies and Health Science, Cardiff and Vale University Health Board, a large integrated organisation commissioning and providing acute, community and tertiary care services. She is also a Director of JJ Consulting Healthcare Management Ltd. Fiona is completing a PhD in management. She is a past Council Member and Vice-President of the Chartered Society of Physiotherapy and a contributor to several Department of Health and NHS Wales working groups.

Fiona and Robert collaboratively lecture both nationally and internationally, lead masterclasses and workshops and give presentations on management and leadership topics and service redesign. They undertake AHP service management reviews and are commissioned for research and surveys. They successfully completed the INSEAD NHS/Leadership Centre Clinical Strategists' Programme at the Business School in Fontainebleau near Paris, and continue to undertake project work with the University. They have both been members of Department of Health working groups on information management and AHP referral to treatment projects. They have a range of publications including the series of *Allied Health Professions Essential Guides*. Their website is: www.jjconsulting.org.uk.

Books in the *Allied Health Professions Essential Guides* Series by Robert Jones and Fiona Jenkins

Developing the Allied Health Professional
ISBN: 9781857757071
2006 Radcliffe Publishing Oxford
www.radcliffehealth.com/shop/developing-allied-health-professional

Managing and Leading in the Allied Health Professions
ISBN: 9781857757064
2006 Radcliffe Publishing Oxford
www.radcliffehealth.com/shop/managing-and-leading-allied-health-professions

Key Topics in Healthcare Management – Understanding the Big Picture
ISBN: 9781857757088
2007 Radcliffe Publishing Oxford
www.radcliffehealth.com/shop/key-topics-healthcare-management-understanding-big-picture

Managing Money, Measurement and Marketing in the AHPs
ISBN: 9781846191985
2010 Radcliffe Publishing Oxford
www.radcliffehealth.com/shop/managing-money-measurement-and-marketing-allied-health-professions

Key Tools and Techniques in Management and Leadership of the Allied Health Professions
ISBN: 9781846195327
2011 Radcliffe Publishing Oxford
www.radcliffehealth.com/shop/key-tools-and-techniques-management-and-leadership-allied-health-professions

Abbreviations

ACPM	Association of Chartered Physiotherapists in Management
AfC	Agenda for Change
AHP	Allied Health Profession
AHPF	Allied Health Professions Federation
AWPM	All Wales Physiotherapy Managers
BDA	British Dietetic Association
BPS	British Psychological Society
CEO	Chief Executive Officer
CfWI	Centre for Workforce Intelligence
CIP	cost improvement programmes
CNO	Chief Nursing Officer
COT	College of Occupational Therapists
CQC	Care Quality Commission
CRES	cash releasing efficiency savings
CSP	Chartered Society of Physiotherapy
DH	Department of Health
DHB	District Health Board
DHSS	Department of Health and Social Security
DNA	did not attend
DRG	diagnosis related group
FTE	full time equivalent
GP	general practitioner
HCA	healthcare assistant
HCPC	Health and Care Professions Council
HPA	Health Policy and Administration
IM&T	Information Management and Technology
ISCP	Irish Society of Chartered Physiotherapists
ITU	Intensive Care/Therapy Unit
LHB	Local Health Board
NHS	National Health Service
NICE	National Institute for Health and Care Excellence
NZ	New Zealand
np	new patient
OT	occupational therapy/therapist
pa	per annum
PDA	personal digital assistant
PT	physical therapist

PTA	physical therapy assistant
RACP	Royal Australian College of Physicians
RCN	Royal College of Nursing
RCP	Royal College of Physicians
RCSLT	Royal College of Speech and Language Therapists
R&D	research and development
RHA	Regional Health Authority
RTT	referral to treatment time
SALT	speech and language therapy
SIGN	Scottish Intercollegiate Guidelines Network
SSA	Safe Staffing Alliance
UK	United Kingdom
UTA	unable to attend
WCPT	World Confederation of Physical Therapy
WHO	World Health Organization
WISN	workload indicators of staffing need
WTE	whole time equivalent

CHAPTER 1

Introduction

Introduction

Following publication early in 2013 of the independent inquiry into serious failings in care provided by the United Kingdom's Mid Staffordshire NHS Foundation Trust, the Francis Report,[1] there has been an increasing recognition that appropriate clinical staffing levels are needed to protect patient safety and provide effective, good quality, compassionate care, respecting patient dignity. For the allied health professions (AHPs) (*see* Appendix 1) this should relate to all areas of service: ward-based, out-patients, community, primary, secondary and tertiary, in all specialties and geographical areas to give assurance that staffing levels are both safe and effective.

Although the main focus on staffing levels nationally has been on nursing services, as a result of the many serious issues set out in the Francis Report,[1] it is clear that patient care requires multidisciplinary and interdisciplinary intervention. There is a risk that staffing numbers in professions such as the AHPs could be significantly reduced, for example, when budgets are under pressure, or during periods of maternity and annual leave, compromising the ability to provide effective treatment and safe care.

For many years it has been recognised within the AHPs that there is need for a robust evidence-based methodology with guidance for the determination of safe and effective staffing levels. In 1991, for example, one of the earliest pieces of work on staffing levels was written and published by the District Physiotherapy Manager for Doncaster Health Authority, Joyce Williams.[2] This booklet arose largely from a series of three workshops which took place in Doncaster in the early 1980s[3-5] and has been the basis of much work that has taken place ever since. However, there is no generally recognised and accepted evidence-based methodology in place for use today. Much staffing levels work throughout the National Health Service (NHS) appears to be based on historical perspectives about what went before, 'rolling the staff establishment over' each year, increasing or decreasing the number of whole time equivalent

(WTE) staff by service redesign and innovation, altering staff establishments almost by estimation or a more or less 'finger in the wind' approach and savings requirements – cost improvement programmes (CIP) and cash releasing efficiency savings (CRES). CRES and CIP are often implemented on an organisation-wide basis where a single percentage resource reduction is required 'across the board' with seemingly little or no analysis of clinical priority and consequent outcomes. It is true that there is some AHP staffing level determination work taking place in a number of locations, but when viewed nationally, this is on a piecemeal basis, hence the need for an evidence-based methodology for determining safe, effective and appropriate staffing levels.

About this book

Important objectives of this book are to support AHP managers and leaders and all those in other disciplines (including service planners, commissioners and policy makers) working on determining staffing levels to facilitate provision of AHP input, to ensure safe care and effective quality outcomes for patients; to report on our review of work done on this issue to date; to give an overview of the national focus on staffing levels in healthcare and to share widely the methodology and supporting tools which we have developed and used.

Staffing level determination is a complex issue which has a crucial bearing on quality service provision. In this book we do not centre on the many elements which comprise quality patient care – this would be a book in itself. However, if our methodology is implemented the resulting staffing levels in different situations and circumstances will ensure that there is the necessary time to facilitate quality care and enable patients to achieve their goals, while providing treatment with compassion, effectiveness and efficiency and respecting dignity.

In Chapter 2 we summarise the impact of important investigations and reports in relation to NHS staffing levels and in Chapter 3 give a flavour of the widespread comment, argument and speculation on NHS staffing levels in the media, indicating the level of public interest. The focus of Chapter 4 is a review of statements, publications and recommendations about NHS staffing levels, providing an overview of any policies and procedures in place and giving a 'feel' for the position of professional bodies and trade unions in healthcare. There is more material available about nursing than any of the other professions, perhaps reflecting that nursing is the largest professional discipline. Medicine and the AHPs are reviewed but there are very few evidence-based policies and recommendations in these professions. International perspectives, particularly in relation to physiotherapy, are also considered in Chapter 4 in order to clarify what we can learn on this topic from other countries.

In Chapter 5 Are there Staffing Level Methodologies for the AHPs?, we report an overview of our scoping work undertaken to investigate whether there is a nationally accepted methodology for determining staffing levels in the NHS AHPs, and to consider various local initiatives and developments over recent decades. As physiotherapy is the largest AHP with a history of some work in this area and as we both have backgrounds in physiotherapy and have managed and led wider AHP services over many years, we used physiotherapy as the case study, but the lessons learned equally apply to the other AHPs.

We present our methodology for determining safe and effective staffing levels for the AHPs in Chapter 6. The processes underpinning our methodology are, firstly, a full assessment of the work which is required to provide a new service, service redesign or review of an existing service: the demand. It is essential that this demand assessment encompasses the many factors which contribute to service quality to ensure that there is enough time for individualised, compassionate care which enables patients to achieve their goals and best possible outcomes. Secondly, calculation and analysis of the 'average' annual activity which can be undertaken by an 'average' staff member (by grading/band and AHP group) and aggregating this figure by the number of staff required to match the demand: capacity. This indicates appropriate evidence-based staffing levels and also incorporates several factors, such as the amount of time available and use of time, throughputs, skill and grade mix, caseload volumes, dependency and costs.

Origins of our approach

Our staffing determination methodology tool has been developed over many years. It is informed by a range of factors and approaches including our experience in AHP management and leadership working nationally and internationally, our work with professional bodies and membership of various Department of Health (DH) and other working groups. The methodology also incorporates elements of methodologies such as that designed and promulgated by Williams,[2] updated for use in healthcare provision today, together with a series of tools and techniques which we have developed, tried and tested and used in our own management and leadership practice. We have conducted many AHP workshops and masterclasses nationally and internationally, and this has enabled us to learn from others and incorporate their ideas into our work. We have undertaken research, scoping and service reviews and have sought information from many sources in the UK and further afield. In order to gain as much information as possible on methods of determining staffing levels in AHP services, we have studied more than 200 publications, contacted at least 30 organisations in the UK and 25 internationally, as well as undertaking 'online' searches. We consider that our methodology is a logical, evidence-based and common sense approach designed to support managers, leaders and all those with responsibility and an interest and who are working in the area of AHP workforce and staffing.

Our methodology will support:

- Evidence-based determination of safe and appropriate staffing levels (workforce design).
- Patient safety.
- Quality service provision and implementation of standards.
- Day-to-day management and leadership and staff deployment.
- Skill mix, case mix work and service model developments.
- Service planning and commissioning.
- Justification of staffing levels.
- Service redesign and innovation.
- Activity analysis and reporting.
- Business cases and cases for change.
- Demand and capacity management.
- Seven day per week service planning.
- Service costing and pricing.
- Resource management.
- Implementation of good quality employment practices.
- Staff learning, development and research and development (R&D).
- Option appraisal.

At the time of publication of this book there is no nationally accepted methodology for undertaking staffing level determination work, nor any guidelines in general use across AHP services. There are no explicit policies or recommendations from professional bodies or Government, although work has taken place on a piecemeal basis for many years. This is a complex area and one that has been the subject of controversy, political 'standpoints' and wide-ranging interest from patients and their representative organisations, the media, the public, professional bodies, trade unions and others from both within and outside the NHS. When we were working on final drafts for this book, the parliamentary Health Select Committee published a third report, *After Francis: Making a Difference*,[6] Section 5 of which covers nursing and healthcare assistant staff in the NHS; clause 141 states:

> *"The standard procedures and practice (for setting fundamental standards) should include evidence-based tools for establishing what each service is likely to require as a minimum in terms of staff numbers and skill mix. This should include nursing staff on wards as well as clinical staff."*

It is not specified which staff groups are included but the term 'clinical staff' generally refers to medical, AHP and other direct patient care staff groups. It continues:

> "These tools should be created after appropriate input from specialties, professional organisations, and patient and public representatives, and consideration for the benefits and value for money of possible staff to patient ratios."

In this book we do not recommend national staffing norms, but rather a practical methodology based on sound calculations derived from the evidence from practice. As Robert Francis put it in his recommendations:

> "To lay down in a regulation 'thou shalt have N number of nurses per patient' is not the answer. The answer is 'how many staff do I need today in this ward to treat these patients?' ... What we need is evidence-based guidance."[1]

Our methodology 'fits' with this approach and demonstrates how it can be done. The Government response indicates that they are not supportive of introducing minimum staffing numbers or ratios on the grounds that this would lead to a lack of flexibility in workforce planning. However, the Government endorses Robert Francis' recommendation that evidence-based guidance should be issued to:

> "inform local decisions on staffing levels, and proposes to work with NICE, CQC [Quality Care Commission] and NHS England to develop such guidance. In reference to the new inspection regime, the CQC will have a remit to inspect staffing levels and to report if wards are inappropriately staffed, and is to require providers to use evidence-based tools to determine staffing numbers."[1]

The full Government response to the Francis Report[1] was published in November 2013.[7] The Government accepted (in full or part) 281 of the 290 recommendations in the report and have asked the National Institute for Health and Care Excellence:

> "to carry out a comprehensive review of the evidence relating to staffing levels in the NHS and to evaluate available relevant data on nursing activities at ward level."[8]

NICE will produce guidance on safe, efficient staffing levels initially focusing on adult wards in acute in-patient settings[8] and then move on to:
- Accident and emergency units.
- Maternity units.
- Acute in-patient paediatric and neonatal wards.
- Mental health in-patient settings.
- Learning disability in-patient units.
- Mental health community units.
- Learning disabilities in the community.
- Community nursing care teams.

Conclusion

Although NICE is only producing guidance about nursing staffing levels, clearly this a much wider NHS issue in the context of safe, effective, quality clinical service provision. The AHPs represent a very significant level of activity providing many millions of patient interventions annually, which are essential to the provision of quality care. Therefore, we believe that now is the right time for work to be undertaken to provide guidance for these essential, wide-ranging and busy services, and this can be achieved through the adoption of a clear methodology; hence the publication of this book at this time.

CHAPTER 2

Key Investigations and Reports

The Francis Report

In February 2013, Robert Francis QC, in his independent inquiry into care failings at the Mid Staffordshire NHS Foundation Trust,[1] recommended that minimum safe staffing levels should be in place. Furthermore, importantly, in his participation at the Care Quality Commission Board meeting on 31 July 2013,[9] he said:

> *"There has been much debate about my recommendations around guidance about staffing levels. So much of what goes wrong in our hospitals is likely, and indeed, to be fair, it was in many regards the case in Mid Stafford, due to there being inadequate staff either in terms of their numbers or skills. And the evidence given to my inquiry was not such as to persuade me however, that there should be a minimum across the board staffing level – I know not everyone agrees with that conclusion, but I could only act on the evidence that I had; I was, after all only dealing with the events arising out of a particular hospital to the inquiry for all its breadth, in the end it had limitations.*
>
> *However, evidence has been put forward to me, certainly since, from the Safe Staffing Alliance to suggest that there is a level below which it should be regarded that a service is not safe, not that that's the adequate level of staffing, but it's a level below which you cannot defect."*

The Francis Report[1] found that a chronic shortage of staff in Mid Staffordshire (particularly nursing) was a major factor in the unacceptably low, seriously substandard care provided, and there have been many renewed calls on Government and healthcare leaders to ensure appropriate levels of staffing on hospital wards to provide proper care and to protect and ensure patient safety.

The Berwick Report

Several further reports and documents have been published since the Francis Report, including, most notably, major reports by Professor Don Berwick[10] and Sir Bruce Keogh, National Medical Director for the NHS in England,[11] as well as the Cavendish Report[12] and documents from the Safe Staffing Alliance (SSA).[13]

Professor Don Berwick, recent advisor to US President Barack Obama, former President of the Institute for Health Improvement and eminent paediatric physician, was requested by the Prime Minister to lead the National Advisory Group in the wake of the Francis Report to report on patient safety in England. *A Promise to Learn – a Commitment to Act: Improving the Safety of Patients in England*[10] was published in July 2013. Berwick covers a wide range of issues on patient safety:

> *"Our job has been to study the various accounts of Mid Staffordshire, as well as the recommendations of Robert Francis and others, to distil for Government and the NHS the lessons learned, and to specify the changes that are needed."*[10]

This is a powerful, succinct and clear report containing a set of essential principles and recommendations. The Berwick Report does not examine what might be adequate or safe staffing levels in depth. However, it does state:

> *"Some of our recommendations have the hard edge of requirement and enforcement. For example, staffing levels should be adequate, based on evidence."*[10]

This recommendation does not specify any particular staff group such as nurses or AHPs; it simply refers to staffing. This is a crucial recommendation, particularly in the light of Francis and others arguing strongly in favour of the necessity for work to be done on staffing levels and then to be acted upon.

The Keogh Report

In February 2013, the Prime Minister and Secretary of State for Health requested Professor Sir Bruce Keogh, KBE conduct a review into the quality of care and treatment provided by hospital Trusts with persistently high mortality rates. This report, *Review into the Quality of Care and Treatment Provided by 14 Hospital Trusts in England: Overview Report*,[11] was predicated on the premise that high mortality rates at Mid Staffordshire NHS Foundation Trust were associated with failure in three dimensions of quality, i.e. clinical effectiveness, patient experience and safety as well as failures in professionalism. This report was not specifically about staffing levels, but focused on safety as one of the important strands; staffing is clearly an integral issue. The review exposed 'fears' over NHS staffing levels, panel members having said that the NHS has little idea whether staffing levels at English hospitals are safe. The report is another part of the jigsaw of evidence leading to the conclusion that work on staffing level determination methodology must be an urgent course of action.

The Cavendish Review

As a result of the findings at the Mid Staffordshire NHS Foundation Trust and failings reported at Winterbourne View, Bristol, the Secretary of State asked Camilla Cavendish (formerly of the *Times* newspaper and now a non-executive director at CQC) to carry out an independent review into healthcare assistants (HCAs) and support workers in the NHS and social care.

According to the Cavendish Review,[12] there are more than 1.3 million front-line non-registered staff working in healthcare, providing care in hospitals, care homes and the homes of individuals. The terms of reference for Camilla Cavendish included recruitment, training, supervision, support and public confidence, but did not include specific reference to staffing levels; however, clearly many of these issues relate directly to safe and adequate staffing levels. The report provided further evidence that staffing levels are an integral part of the overall pattern, and that many of the issues cannot be successfully addressed and resolved without attention to ensuring adequate staffing throughout the service through relevant, effective methodologies and tools.

Wales, Scotland and Northern Ireland

Although the Francis Report[1] and many of the reviews that followed in the wake of Francis have been explicitly about NHS organisations in England, the issues are also relevant to NHS services in Wales, Scotland and Northern Ireland. There have been several media reports about substandard healthcare provision in some organisations within the three countries and the issue has been the subject of discussion, accompanied by calls for action. The issue is also under discussion at Government level within Northern Ireland, Scotland and Wales.

The Welsh Government has discussed the issue in some detail. The National Assembly for Wales Research Services[14] provides a summary table of nurse staffing levels in Local Health Boards (LHBs) in Wales, which demonstrates wide discrepancies in staffing. It states:

> "The final report of the inquiry into failings in the Mid Staffordshire NHS Foundation Trust found that a chronic shortage of staff, particularly nursing staff, was a major factor in the substandard care provided."

In her response to the Francis Report, the then Welsh Health Minister, Lesley Griffiths AM, set out a number of action points including plans to introduce a new assessment process to determine staffing levels on wards, based on severity of patients' conditions – 'acuity' rather than solely patient numbers:[15]

> "In the interim, the NHS (in Wales) is using a core set of principles to determine staffing levels on all medical and surgical wards."

The principles referred to were developed by the Chief Nursing Officer (CNO) in Wales and issued to all Health Boards in Wales in 2012. The principles included:

> "The number of patients per registered nurse should not exceed 7 by day."

The skill mix of registered nurses to nursing support worker in acute areas should generally be 60:40; however, the staffing levels quoted in the Welsh Research Services Note[14] indicate staffing levels which are at considerable variance to this. On 17 April 2013, Wales' Health Minister, Mark Drakeford AM, said, in answer to a question whether he would support statutory minimum staffing levels:[16a]

> "That is a proposition to which I will give thought. ... Whether the most sensible way to proceed is to then embed that in legislation is a question that is, I think, worth considering, and I will give it that consideration."

The CNO for Wales has developed a 'tool' that will respond to rapidly changing clinical situations. Professor Jean White CNO told the National Assembly's Health and Social Care Committee that Health Boards had been working to action plans for staffing levels. She said:

> "I think there is danger in setting any kind of thing that is a blanket set of principles as there needs to be a judgement."

In a plenary session of the Welsh Government in March 2014[16b] a vote took place and it was agreed that work should be sanctioned to develop nurse staffing levels, but there was no indication when the work was scheduled to be completed. This resulted from introduction of a Member Proposed Bill by Kirsty Williams AM, on minimum nurse staffing levels.

> "This Legislation would require the Government to produce regulations which set a minimum staffing level for nurses in Wales. These regulations would be required to set minimum nurse staffing levels for each different acute and specialist service. I am also mindful to include a requirement for the regulations to address the complexity of patients' needs and on the skills mix in a hospital. The Legislation would also give the Government the power to issue similar regulations for community nursing, but only when they considered that sufficient evidence exists to support regulations in this area. There is increasing evidence from across the world that having more nurses per patient substantially improves the care

> received by patients in the NHS. Most recently the Francis Report cited long-term low staffing levels as one reason which contributed to poor treatment".[1]
>
> Similar legislation has been introduced in California, New South Wales and Victoria (Australia) where it has improved nurse staffing levels and patient care. Studies in California have shown that minimum levels are effective in increasing staffing levels and in reducing mortality rates. Emerging evidence from Australia suggests that this is true there as well."[16b]

In Scotland, the Scottish Government announced in November 2012[17] that from 2013:

> "Nurse and midwife staffing levels in Scottish hospitals will be set using mandatory workforce planning tools."

Other comment and conclusion

The SSA, an organisation set up in 2012 which includes the Royal College of Nursing, The Patients' Association, the Florence Nightingale Foundation and the trade union UNISON, states that wards regularly have one registered nurse caring for eight patients, a ratio which they say is "*unsafe*".[13] They argue that this ratio should not be regarded as a minimum acceptable level of staffing, and say research has shown the risk of harm and death increases if a nurse is asked to look after more than eight patients.

According to a BBC News Report,[18] Health Minister Dan Poulter stated:

> "The soon-to-be appointed chief inspector of hospitals would be tasked with taking action if hospitals were found to be compromising patient care by not having the right number of staff on the wards."

In their report *Compassion in Practice, Nursing, Midwifery and Care Staff: our Vision and Strategy, 2012*[19] the NHS Commissioning Board states that to:

> "deliver the vision, we need the right number of staff with the right skills and behaviour and working in the right place to meet the needs of the people they are for."

This is a well worn phrase, but nevertheless an important declaration of intent. The strategy states that local organisations can support by:

> "ensuring that Boards sign off and publish evidence-based staffing levels at least every 6 months, linked to quality of care and patient experience and discuss this in Public Board meetings",[19]

with commissioners reviewing the staffing levels using evidence-based tools/

methodology linking with quality and patient experience and ensuring appropriate action is taken.

Although this document is aimed specifically at nursing, midwifery and care staff we argue that the sentiments which it expresses should be applied to all professional groups providing clinical services across the whole of the NHS. Taken together with the reports published during 2013, the Government response, the high level of pressure from patient representative organisations, professional and trade union bodies, the media and the public at large, it would appear that work on staffing level determination methodology is imminent at national level and, therefore, it is the right time and opportunity for a strategy and action plan to be put in place for AHP staffing level determination.

CHAPTER 3

Media Focus and Reporting

The Francis Report[1] found that a chronic shortage of staff in Mid Staffordshire – particularly nursing – was a major factor in the unacceptably low, seriously substandard care provided, and there have been many calls on Government and healthcare leaders to ensure appropriate levels of staffing on hospital wards to provide proper care and to protect and ensure patient safety.

Nurse staffing levels in the UK are set at local level by individual provider organisation Boards of Directors and this is also true for the AHPs.

Since publication of the Francis report[1] there has been a plethora of news items and articles appeared in the media calling for work to be put in place to determine and ensure safe staffing levels, appropriate skill mix and a methodology for calculating safe and evidence-based staffing. Some have also argued that staffing level guidance should be made mandatory. However, we do not support this stance as staffing levels need to be determined in line with many factors such as patient dependency, different specialties, local circumstances and so on.

A random 'snapshot' of just a few of the many articles and media coverage headlines over the summer of 2013 gives a flavour of the wide interest and comment:

> *"Jeremy Hunt urged to set NHS safe staffing levels after Mid Staffs scandal – Minimum safe staffing levels were recommended 6 months ago by Robert Francis in his review of catastrophic care failings at the Mid Staffordshire NHS Trust."*[20]

> *"One in ten nurses fears a repeat of Mid Staffs where they work. Almost half of nurses believe their ward has the wrong skill mix, Nursing Standard has found ... Our UK-wide poll of nearly 1,700 nurses revealed concerns over staffing levels and patient care."*[21]

> *"The case for increased nurse staffing levels – Given the imperative of keeping patients safe in hospital, it certainly makes sense to approach the challenge of setting staffing levels in a more analytical and systematic way than has been the case in the past."*[22]

"Nurses condemn unsafe staffing levels – Senior nurses have issued an unprecedented warning about hospital ward staffing levels in England. The Safe Staffing Alliance, which includes the RCN, says wards regularly have one registered nurse caring for eight patients, which is unsafe. ... The warning follows a study by researchers at Southampton University, King's College London and the National Nursing Research Unit."[23]

"Daytime staffing levels must never fall below 1 to 8, says expert group – Florence Nightingale Foundation said: 'If staffing exceeds a ratio of one registered nurse to eight patients, there is a significantly increased risk of harm.'"[24]

"Staffing levels, who's counting? – With the Keogh review highlighting the link between low staffing levels and outcomes, patient to nurse ratios are again in the spotlight ... This issue of staffing and outcomes is more complex than instigating ratios would suggest."[25]

"Hospital watchdog warns 17 organisations have unsafe staffing levels – Care Quality Commission says inspections show facilities and staff are not enough to 'keep people safe'."[26]

"The Chair of the Mid Staffordshire Foundation Trust Public Inquiry has called for a rethink on minimum nurse staffing levels – less than 6 months after deciding not to recommend mandatory ratios in his landmark report. Robert Francis QC last week suggested to regulators that a minimum staffing level should act as an 'alarm bell' for questions about safety, in the same way as high mortality rates. In February, nursing unions and other campaigners had been disappointed Mr. Francis did not go further on staffing levels. ... Although he called for nationally recognised tools for establishing appropriate staffing levels, he stopped short of backing the introduction of mandatory minimum nurse-to-patient ratios.

However, during a public appearance last week, Mr. Francis said he had seen evidence from the SSA – a confederation of nursing and patient groups set up earlier this year – that had convinced him the issue should be revisited. 'It's evidence that ought to be considered with regard to whether there is some sort of benchmark, which at least is a bit like mortality rates – ... .' He stressed the level should not be viewed as 'the adequate level of staffing, but the level below which you cannot be safe'."[27]

Sally Brearley, Chair of the Prime Minister's forum on Nursing and Care Quality, said a

"pivotal moment in the debate on minimum nurse staffing levels had now been reached."[27]

There have been scores of reports in the media and medical press throughout 2013 of which these examples are typical, indicating the pressure building for work to be commenced at national level on the staffing levels issue within the NHS. In the Readers' comment section of the same *Health Service Journal* publication[27] it was reported that Jim Buchan, Professor of Health Sciences at Edinburgh Queen Margaret University, said:

> "The lack of progress was surprising ... They are not even at the starting block yet, it doesn't feel like minimum staffing is something that is going to go away. This is a significant job which would require a lot of resources ... it's not something that will be achieved overnight ... we need tools that are relevant to the care environment."

Roger Kline said.

> "The evidence is even clearer now as the excellent work done by the Staffing Alliance and others shows, and as Robert Francis recently acknowledged."[28,29]

The content of investigation reports and studies discussed in Chapter 2 demonstrates why the wide range of media coverage, comment and speculation relates to nursing staffing levels. However, the NHS is now at a point where not to include work on AHP and other patient care staffing levels would be a serious lost opportunity.

CHAPTER 4

Where do the Professions Stand? Statements, Publications and Recommendations

The main focus of this chapter is a scoping of statements, publications and recommendations from key professional organisations – nursing, medicine and the AHPs – together with information obtained from international physiotherapy professional bodies. However, the AHP section in this chapter does not include physiotherapy – the largest of the AHPs in the UK – as this is discussed in a case study section in Chapter 5.

Nursing

The National Nursing Research Unit, King's College London[30] notes some concerns in their *Overview of Research Evidence*:

> *"Registered nurse staffing levels vary considerably in English hospitals. In some NHS hospitals registered nurses will provide care to an average of five named patients during a shift, whilst in other hospitals the nurses have up to 11 patients to care for. While a degree of variation in staffing between units is expected and necessary because of differences in patient needs and the type of care provided, research has found considerable variation between and within hospitals even when specialty and patient dependency are controlled for. Some wards can be well staffed while other wards are dangerously understaffed.*
>
> *… When the numbers are added up across a hospital the overall staffing levels can appear to be adequate. Planning safe nurse staffing levels is a recognised problem in many countries, … and the UK Care Quality Commission Reports consistently warn that quality and staffing vary considerably within NHS hospitals. Neglected care (or care not done because of time pressures) is correlated to low registered nurse staffing on the ward.*
>
> *… Under-staffing has cost implications for hospitals. Emergency admissions*

are higher where there are few registered nurses and nurses are likely to suffer more injuries and stress, exacerbating staffing problems and costs.
  … Some specialties – such as old people's care – typically suffer lower staffing levels and more dilute skill mix. Fifty per cent of the nursing workforce caring for older people is made up of care assistants.
  … Internationally the research evidence to show that nurse staffing levels have an impact on patient outcomes is substantial."

It is asserted in the SSA Statement of May 2013[13] that:

"Given the compelling evidence of a link between registered nurse levels and the quality of care, the SSA believes that endeavours to ensure compassionate care must be underpinned by adequate nurse staffing levels if they are to succeed."

The SSA recommends:[13]

"1. Planning for nurse staffing on wards is undertaken in every ward in every Trust, supported by evidence-based tools/methodologies to set core establishments sufficient to maintain safe nurse to patient ratios.
2. Ward sisters (or equivalent) are empowered to make day-to-day decisions on staffing and resource levels with the authority to act on those decisions.
3. Ward sisters and nurse managers are supported by the Director of Nursing and the Trust Board; the Trust Board must be accountable for staffing levels being maintained at the calibrated safe and appropriate levels.
4. Under no circumstances is it safe to care for patients in need of hospital treatment with a ratio of more than 8 patients per registered nurse during the day time on general acute wards including those specialising in care for older people.
5. If registered nurse staffing falls below a ratio of 1 nurse to 8 patients (excluding the nurse in charge) it is a requirement that this be reported and recorded; there is evidence that risk of harm to patients is substantially increased at these staffing levels.
6. Trusts are required to report the frequency of such incidents publicly and to take immediate action to remedy the breach. If breaches occur regularly this must be escalated through the Trust's risk management systems.
7. Registered nurses must at all times be supported by a sufficient number of healthcare assistants and a senior registered nurse in charge of the ward."

In summary, the main thrust of the argument is that where staffing levels are low care is compromised; in situations where there is an excessive number of patients per registered nurse, there is an associated higher than expected mortality rate and *"other harms"*. The document states[13] that 1:8 is the level *at which care is considered to be unsafe*; it is not a recommended minimum.
  The recommendations set out in the SSA statement[13] are based on multiple

sources of evidence.[31-37] The Research Evidence notes[30] and the SSA statement[13] also argue for the use of evidence-based tools and methodologies to set core nursing establishments. Research undertaken through Southampton University by Peter Griffiths and colleagues from the National Nursing Research Unit, published by the British Medical Journal's *Quality and Safety Journal*[38] also reports powerful research on the current state of nursing staffing levels.

Discussion, debate and work about staffing levels in nursing is not new; for some years the development of methodologies, approaches and tools has been taking place. In 2010, for example, the Royal College of Nursing (RCN) published *RCN Policy Position: Evidence-based Nurse Staffing Levels*.[39] This wide-ranging policy position covered a number of important areas including outcome measurement, skill mix, dependency, pressure to identify 'optimum nurse staffing levels', how staffing levels should be determined and so on. Although positive that the RCN published this document in 2010, it did not, however, move the NHS much nearer to identifying a specific way forward.

In March 2012 the RCN published a policy briefing: *Mandatory Nurse Staffing Levels*.[37] The RCN argued that mandatory nurse staffing levels would provide an important guarantee for patients during *"this challenging period"*. This document was set in a framework where nurse staffing levels were determined locally by individual healthcare providers. These local arrangements include both the number of patients per nurse and the number of registered nurses to unregistered healthcare support staff, and the mix and experience of registered nursing staff. The DH in England and professional organisations – including the RCN – have produced a range of guidance outlining recommended staffing levels for some care settings. However, there is no *"compliance regime, or compulsion on providers to follow these when planning services"*.[37]

Mandatory Nurse Staffing Levels is an informative and useful overview of the staffing levels situation, clearly highlighting many facets of this complex issue. The document summarises the case for introducing a system of mandatory safe staffing levels based on:

> *"The growing body of evidence which shows that nurse staffing levels make a difference to outcomes …*
> *… Successive reports into care failings have highlighted the risks associated with employing too few nursing staff …*
> *… Despite a number of research studies showing the correlation between higher nurse staffing levels and the improved care outcomes, RCN members continue to report lower nurse-to-patient ratios than research suggests is safe …*
> *… Financial challenges and global economic downturn are leading to higher numbers of nursing posts being cut and concerns exist over a significant dilution of the workforce …"*[37]

The policy document is specifically nursing oriented; however, the history outlined, reference to the plethora of reports, papers, methodologies, tools and arguments – together with an international perspective – form part of a strong argument for work to be done on staffing levels determination without further delay.

For Northern Ireland:[40]

> "The Government has announced that in Northern Ireland a review of nursing staffing levels will be set up as part of a three year workforce plan.
> ... The Northern Ireland Health Minister – Edwin Poots – has asked the Department of Health, Social Services and Public Safety and Chief Nursing Officer – to draw up the plan. The use of skill mix within nursing teams will be investigated together with the use of nursing staff deployed through 'banks' and agencies, the work will also include the provision of nurse education and training."

In Scotland, standardised workforce planning tools are in place across the NHS. In addition, standards exist that cover inspections of the social care sector and NHS wards. These are currently under review.[37]

In Wales, the LHBs undertake workforce planning in the context of Welsh Government guidance and oversight. Individual LHBs set their own staffing establishments as workforce planning is localised. There is *"significant variation in workforce models across NHS organisations in Wales"*.[37] The issue is recognised by the Welsh Government and:

> "It is likely that it will make a commitment in the future through a new human resources and organisational Development Framework to improving the situation, making more explicit workforce planning arrangements and addressing variations in workforce models across the NHS in Wales."[37]

Planning Nurse Staffing Levels on Acute Wards in Wales, a report prepared by the Wales Professional Nurse Staffing Group[41] argues that Wales *"needs to take a pro-active approach to the management and deployment of its nursing workforce based on a sound evidence-base, data and information"*. This document sets out a brief review of relevant literature.

One example from the literature about staffing levels, skill mix, outcomes and other relevant topic areas aimed at supporting a methodical approach to staffing level determination for nursing is *Safe Staffing for Older People's Wards, an RCN Toolkit*.[42] This represents just one of the many toolkits and methodologies available and in use in some geographical areas and in some specialty areas in nursing.

The five most common toolkits or workforce planning methods in use in the UK within nursing were presented in a paper published by the RCN Policy Unit in September 2006, *Setting Appropriate Ward Nurse Staffing Levels in NHS Acute Trusts*.[43] The policy guidance draws together:

- Research evidence linking registered nurse numbers and expertise to patient outcomes.
- Data on nursing workforce and nursing staffing levels.
- Methods available for setting nurse staffing levels.
- Discussion about setting nurse to patient ratios.

This document details guidance and principles advising on how to review ward staffing levels including the recommendation that a:

> "benchmark ward establishment skill-mix ratio is set out, 65% registered nurses to 35% health care assistants unless or until a thorough staffing review is undertaken in accordance with RCN principles."

The RCN Policy Unit asserted that nursing staffing levels matter.

> "because of the evidence that links patient outcomes to registered nurse input, staff morale, staff turnover and job dissatisfaction."

In common with Francis, Berwick, Keogh and Cavendish,[1,10-12] nurse staffing levels were, at the time of publication of this policy guidance (2006), seen as a:

> "patient safety issue ... and it should be accepted that human interventions are at least as important as technologies such as drugs, devices and techniques in health outcomes and so require an equally robust evidence-based and commensurate research funding."

This policy guidance also clearly states that:

> "Many hospitals do not have a systematic approach to choosing or using methods to review ward staffing levels and there is no agreement about the 'best' tool to use."

It is asserted that "essentially there are two different approaches". Firstly, measuring nurse staffing levels and their impact on outcomes for patients, staff and the provider organisations, and, secondly, measuring what staff actually do. As a basis for a methodology for calculating safe staffing levels, these two approaches appear limited as measuring current staffing levels and their impact on outcomes does not indicate a level for staffing, but merely identifies some of the issues. Measuring what staff actually do is only part of the picture, because in order to develop a robust methodology it is necessary to measure annual average capacity and use of time rather than only looking at what is done.

The document concludes with an overview of the five most common workforce planning methods used in nursing, at the time of its publication. The systems examined in Appendix 3 to the RCN document were:

- Professional judgement approach.
- Nurse per occupied bed method.
- Acuity-quality method.
- Timed-task/activity approaches.
- Regression-based systems.

All of these methods have their advantages and disadvantages, but none of them explores what might be the available work/activity capacity of a nurse throughout a period of time, which could then be aggregated to give potential service capacity data for a ward, section, specialty, department, hospital, taking into account patient dependency, specialty and so on.

The approaches examined in the RCN Policy Unit document are not appropriate for the AHP services because none of the approaches provides a complete picture.

Together with Francis,[1] Berwick,[10] Keogh[11] and Cavendish,[12] the specific statements, publications and recommendations directly from the nursing profession indicate that work on safe staffing levels needs to progress rapidly. Even though the approach in nursing is not consistent 'across the board' in the UK or even throughout any of the four countries individually, the case is well made for a coherent approach to a methodology for determining safe staffing levels, skill mix relative to dependency, outcomes and other parameters to be put in place.

Medical services

To obtain as broad a picture as possible of how staffing levels are determined and whether there are robust methodologies and processes in place for this across a wide spectrum of NHS services, we contacted several medical, surgical and other Royal Colleges to request any information they had on safe staffing levels. Very little information was available; however, some useful background information was obtained from the Royal College of Physicians (RCP) which is outlined here.

The RCP document *Setting Higher Standards: Consultant Physicians Working with Patients; the Duties, Responsibilities and Practice of Physicians in Medicine*[44] makes a number of references to workforce planning, but, in common with other medical organisations, does not specify any particular method or process for their determination. However, the points of concern they mentioned indicate that staffing levels are important and an area in which development work should take place.

> "... over the past few years with the creation of the Centre for Workforce Intelligence (CfWI) to replace the Workforce Review Team. This organisation is an information source to allow workforce planning locally, but despite good intention there remains considerable anxiety about the quality of the data on the current workforce, let alone the models used to plan the future workforce ... The

medical specialties, the RCP and the CfWI need to work together over the next few years to ensure that uniform data are used and that sensible predictions are made to plan training numbers.

The workload of the medical registrar has become very heavy and changes need to be made to have more doctors on the wards and dealing with the emergency intake."[44]

In a document entitled *Patient Safety Policy*[45] the RCP states:

"Poor service design introduces a number of barriers to the provision of appropriate, high quality care centred around needs of the patient. Health and social care professionals need to be supported by a system designed to promote the delivery of high quality care. Existing evidence tells us that the following need to be in place: adequate staffing numbers, with sufficient time available to care for patients."

This is also stated by the RCP in *Commission in Improving Dignity in Care for Older People*,[46] in 2011. In commenting on the Berwick Report[10] the RCP stated:

"An emphasis on appropriate staffing levels would also help the NHS cope with the increasing strain it is under due to the inexorable rise in emergency admissions ... "[47]

While these RCP papers do not add 'hard' evidence about methodologies for the determination of appropriate staffing levels, together with the anecdotal evidence available from other doctors' organisations, it is clear that staffing levels, skill mix, workforce planning, patient safety, qualified to assistant staff ratios and kindred issues are of great concern to them and that they support the thrust of the major reports which were published during 2013.[1,10–12]

Allied health professions

As we are Chartered Physiotherapists ourselves with established access to the Chartered Society of Physiotherapy (CSP) staff and colleagues throughout the profession, as well as working closely with CSP on management and leadership topics, we used our established links to ascertain whether there was any physiotherapy guidance available officially from the professional body on safe and effective staffing levels. The CSP had no formal policy or guidance, but we discuss a wide range of background material from a variety of sources in our case study in Chapter 5.

In order to gain access to other AHP colleagues, we contacted the Allied Health Professions Federation (AHPF) administration and representatives from 12 of the professional bodies in the Federation, with the exception of physiotherapy. A response was received from AHPF administration which stated that staffing levels were not "*something the AHPF can help with*", together with a suggestion to contact the professional bodies themselves. Of these 12 only five organisations responded.

All five organisations said that queries about staffing levels were "*coming up frequently*". One had contacted the Workforce Review Team and the Professional Officers at the DH and it soon became obvious that:

> "*There are no figures for this held nationally at the DH.*
> *Far from being an exact science, it is calculated more or less on the basis of what is provided at present, combined with an estimation of what should be provided.*"[48]

The British Dietetic Association (BDA) published a paper several years ago on workload management and have recently made available some comparison figures:

> "*These were determined by a variety of different methodologies, mostly audits and pragmatic approaches, e.g. if this is a service model, how many dietitians/ support workers do you think it will need to … ?*"[49]

The College of Occupational Therapists (COT)[50] pointed out that the "*area of predicting staffing levels*" can present problems:

> "*Where a service for whatever reason has more than the recommended number of occupational therapists (OTs) it has been used in evidence to reduce staffing numbers.*"

The COT also clarified that OTs work in significant numbers in social care organisations as well as in the NHS and also, like physiotherapy, cover all four nations in the UK. They maintain that there is a "*need in some areas for greater numbers of occupational therapists*" which could be "*predicted by geography and prevalence of certain conditions. All these matters present problems when setting a standard for numbers of professional staff per head of population.*"[50] The COT had worked closely with the Centre for Workforce Intelligence (CfWI) in "*terms of predicting need for future workforce and developed assumptions*". They also drew attention to the work of the CfWI.

The Royal College of Speech and Language Therapists (RCSLT) drew attention to their document *Calculating Hours Available to a FTE Speech and Language Therapist*,[51] which is based on the work of Joyce Williams.[2]

The AHP professional bodies said that they are under a lot of pressure to provide information and guidance on staffing levels for their members and others and that only limited advice is provided by them. There is no recognised national methodology. All organisations responding to the request for information expressed interest in this work and asserted that work needs to be done without delay on developing a methodology for determining safe and appropriate staffing levels.

There are many documents relevant to the AHPs, generally produced by the professional bodies and their specific clinical interest groups, providing evidence on the effectiveness of their services and the types of interventions and modalities. These generally, however, lack detailed information on the intensity or quantity of treatment or staffing levels required to achieve the desired outcomes. It is clear that any guidance on staffing levels required in specific areas needs to relate to skill mix, case mix and desired or anticipated outcomes. No consistent methodology or guidance is in place for use across the AHPs or NHS as a whole.

An example of the guidance and recommendations available includes the *National Clinical Guideline for Stroke* by the Intercollegiate Stroke Working Party.[52] This document contains more than 300 recommendations covering many aspects of stroke management. Specific recommendations on staffing levels and skill mix are not developed, but many aspects of quality, audit, training and staff availability are included, in addition to specific sections on wide ranging aspects of clinical care, and many other topics. The document sets out detailed recommendations on what services should be provided by:

- Consultant physicians.
- Nurses.
- Physiotherapists.
- OTs.
- Speech and language therapists.
- Dietitians.
- Clinical psychologists.
- Social workers.

It also includes reference to education programmes for all staff providing the stroke service including 'junior professionals' and access to pharmacy, orthotics, orthoptists, specialist seating, patient information advice and support and assistive devices. It advises that each acute stroke unit should have immediate access to medical staff specially trained in acute medical care for stroke patients, imaging and laboratory services and rehabilitation specialist staff.

> *"Each stroke rehabilitation unit and service should be organised as a single team of staff with specialist knowledge and experience of stroke and neurological rehabilitation."*[52]

The document has little advice about staffing levels and no advice about methodologies for determining these. However, in setting out detailed information, advice and recommendations about the roles, duties and functions of the rehabilitation team as a collaborative unit, it paves the way for thinking about possible staffing levels in terms of clinical pathway development, as well as what staffing is needed by the individual clinical professions as component parts of integrated clinical teams.

For recommendations on actual staffing levels the RCP advice emanating from the Sentinel audits[53] is widely known within the AHPs. This sets out the whole time equivalents (WTE) staff on stroke units. The data are presented as ratios of staff per 10 stroke unit beds.

Other documents specifically about stroke services[54–56] indicate figures for staffing levels. Figures are set out for each of the professions in stroke rehabilitation units. The numbers are benchmarks provided through the Sentinel audit;[53] they are not based on a specific calculation methodology.

The Concise Guides for Stroke 2012 are profession-specific concise guidelines for each of the professions involved. The NHS Quality Improvement Scotland, The Scottish Intercollegiate Guidelines Network (SIGN) also sets out recommendations for staffing levels in *Management of Patients with Stroke: Rehabilitation, Prevention and Management of Complications, and Discharge Planning – a National Clinical Guideline*[57] but, in common with many other publications, there is no indication about the methodology for their determination.

Although there are a number of publications about staffing levels for integrated multidisciplinary teams quoting various audits which have taken place at national or local levels (for example, the RCP Sentinel audit),[53] it is arguable that the individual component professional clinical parts of the whole will need to lay down certain specifications about what constitutes safe and acceptable staffing levels, qualified to non-qualified staff ratios, grade and skill mix and so on. There is a range of documents published by various organisations which do not quote methodologies or figures for specific staffing (for example, for speech and language therapy).[58–65]

For clinical psychology services, the British Psychological Society (BPS) in *Briefing Paper 5: Commissioning Clinical Psychology Services for Older People, their Families and other Carers*, 2006[66] recommended minimum staffing levels for a *"typical district service population of 250,000 of which around 45,000 will be more than 65 years of age – one WTE clinical psychologist per 10,000 older people"*. However, the document concedes that the recommendations will need to be adjusted according to local needs, taking into account factors such as local indices of deprivation and age profiles. Recommendations are also given for secondary mental health services for older people. Staffing levels for primary care psychology may be calculated in various ways depending on the model adopted by local services.[67]

Other recommendations are given for young onset dementia services, stroke services, falls services and intermediate care. However, a methodology for determination of staffing levels is not explained.

A somewhat different approach is adopted in *Guidance for Best Practice: the Employment of Counsellors and Psychotherapists in the NHS*.[68] Here, the British Association of Clinical Psychologists recommend 2 hours of counselling per 1000 population for low-deprivation localities and 4.5 hours per 1000 population for high-deprivation localities, but the methodology for supporting this recommendation is not given.

In summary, there are many documents and guidelines about the roles, standards, effectiveness, treatments and benefits available, and the advice and care provided by AHPs, but there is little, if any, robust evidence-based information on the intensity of treatment or staffing levels required to obtain the desired outcomes or information about methodologies for determining them.

An international perspective

We conducted an international case study about physiotherapy staffing levels and any methodologies for determining these. To this end, the Authors contacted the Head Office of the World Confederation of Physical Therapy (WCPT) to ascertain whether they were aware of any information or work on safe staffing levels from member organisations. They were unable to provide any information, but recommended contacting a sample of the individual professional organisations around the world. The names and addresses of the chief executive officers (CEOs) and organisations of the WCPT European CEOs Forum were obtained and supplemented with others more widely to obtain as broad a coverage as possible. Personal contacts were also made with colleagues internationally. Altogether, 25 physiotherapy/physical therapy professional bodies around the globe were contacted. Of these, 13 countries responded but most of them were unable to provide any information or documentation. However, all were interested in the work which they saw as very important.

At the time of writing, information for Luxembourg is not available but *"our Health Minister is trying to determine the staffing number in his next 'Plan Hospitalier'".*[69] In Norway, there are currently no statutory requirements for the number of physiotherapists in any healthcare sector, and the Norwegian health authorities have not made staffing recommendations. The only *"Domain"* where work has taken place on this is in school health services, where in a 2010 study by the Norwegian Directorate of Health[70] they stipulated a ratio of just over one full-time position per 1600 pupils *"a 56 percent physiotherapist per 800 pupils to be precise"* – 0.56 WTE per 800 pupils. *"However, this norm did not become part of the new Health and Care Services Act, which took effect on 1.1.2012."*[70]

The position in Ireland is:

> *"The Workforce Planning and Business Group of the Irish Society of Chartered Physiotherapists (ISCP) has been convened in recent years to address a range of issues including WTE resources requirements/productivity expectations. The group hopes to develop Irish consensus recommendations on staffing ratios and anticipates finalising and publishing/circulating this element of its work remit over the next year or so."*[71]

In Germany there is no particular formula or methodology for determining how many physiotherapists each hospital should have relative to the number of beds – neither in hospitals nor in the private practice sector in which outpatients are treated.

> *"Every hospital in Germany has to set up their own budget. The reimbursement system is based on the diagnoses related group system (DRGs). That means that the hospital will get a certain amount of funding for any individual case. The amount is negotiated by the National Hospital Association and the Association of the National Health Insurance Providers on an annual basis. In the calculation of the flat rate per case every service is included (so, also physiotherapy). The calculation itself is secret.*
>
> *Out-patients are treated in private practice. There are no regulations about how many physiotherapists in an area/town are allowed to treat in a private practice, but opening a private physiotherapy practice has to fulfil a list of regulations laid down in the national agreement negotiated between the national body and the Association of the National Health Insurance Providers."*[72]

The funding for physiotherapy services in the private sector is analysed annually through the social health insurances. How much money is spent on physiotherapy is prescribed.

From Physiotherapy New Zealand (NZ) there is:

> *"No formula for determining what staffing levels should be ... trying to see what the average staffing levels were and the individual hospitals could see if they were close to the average. Some have used the data to argue for increased staffing in a specific clinical area.*
>
> *The latest information on staffing levels is based on a 2010 survey ... responsibility has shifted to the Registration Board."*[73]

The NZ response continues:

> *"This is a fascinating study and it will hopefully provide some information that many physiotherapists are grappling with ... in the past we have done some brief surveys of our public hospitals (DHBs) to try and establish a benchmark for staffing levels, it has always been fraught with difficulties as case mixes vary so much between hospitals."*[73]

It is interesting to note that the NZ physiotherapy workforce is currently 3915 physiotherapists with 'current practicing certificates' serving a population of 4,468,000.

Approximately one-third of the workforce are employed in the public sector system and others in private practice or other areas such as schools, research and teaching. Approximately 1300 physiotherapists are employed in the public sector for a population just a little higher than the population of Wales.

From the United States the reviewers obtained an article *PT to PTA Staffing Levels – What is the Community Standard?*.[74] This article provided a commentary on the Health Policy and Administration (HPA) 'Burning Question' for June 2012 which focused on physical therapy assistant (PTA) to physical therapist (PT) ratios. The HPA 'Burning Question' polls the physical therapy community on hot topics on a regular basis. There is very little in the literature regarding staffing ratios; this, the only information we could find specifically about staffing level issues in the AHPs in the United States search, stated:

> "... Many clinical leaders are looking at their most valuable yet expensive resource, their staffs and re-evaluating the mix of PTAs to Physiotherapist (PTs) ... given the realities of the marketplace, for those questioning their mix of PTAs to PTs, there is likely the desire to know what the community standard is for the ratio of PTAs to PTs. Many States have in their physical therapy practice Acts, provision restricting the number of PTAs any one PT can supervise, but the question is if PT clinics are staffing at those ratios or if they are doing something different."

The purpose of the 'Burning Question' poll was to gather data about the ratio of PTAs to PTs in clinical practice, to be able to give clinical leaders information about current standards in the community as a whole. This was undertaken in the light of growing pressure to reduce costs across the entire healthcare sector. *"It is important for physical therapy leaders to know the current community standard for PTA usage."*[74]

The poll found:
- 37% of respondents were in in-patient settings.
- 52% were in out-patient settings.
- 4% in home health.
- 7% in other.
- The average staffing ratio for all clinics in all settings was 1 PTA to every 4 PTs (169 PTAs to 728 PTs), i.e. 19% of total staff members were PTAs. However, this was a relatively small survey with only 95 respondents.

The ratio of physiotherapy assistants to graduate staff was also a topic investigated in a NZ study.[75] The NZ survey showed a range from six physiotherapists to one assistant to two physiotherapists to one assistant. The latter was due to staffing shortages where three overseas physiotherapists had been employed as assistants while waiting for their registration to be finalised and was an outlier.

A document published by the Royal Australian College of Physicians and Australasian Faculty of Rehabilitation Medicine (2011) entitled *Standards for the Provision of Adult Rehabilitation Medicine Services in Public and Private Hospitals*[76] was made available to us. It states:

> *"The purpose of these standards is to guide Royal Australian College of Physicians (RACP) fellows, Government, Health Service planners and administrators in their decision making about the provision of an adult in-patient rehabilitation medicine service in public and private hospitals ... the document incorporates up-dated best practice guidelines into one single document which can be used as a reference ... Many of the standards are expressed as consensus statements of good rehabilitation practice."*

With regard to rehabilitation medicine the document states:

> *"Allied Health Staff ... Patients will receive an appropriate quantum and mix of therapy to enable them to achieve an optimal rehabilitation outcome within an appropriate timeframe. This will vary according to individual patient facts ... there is mounting evidence in the literature on the benefits of greater therapy intensity in improving functional outcomes and improving the efficiency of the rehabilitation process."*

It is asserted that the appropriate amount of therapy that patients receive will range from a minimum of 3 hours for patients who have the *"capacity to tolerate this amount of therapy, down to lesser amounts, based on patient need and capacity to participate"*.[76] AHP staff to patient ratios for each 10 patients are set out in a table which includes figures for physiotherapy in amputation, stroke/neurology, orthopaedics, major trauma, spinal cord dysfunction, traumatic brain injury, pain and reconditioning and restorative. There are, for example, clauses on:
- Adjustment of staffing levels to suit case mix.
- Adjustment of staffing levels to account for time spent doing other things than patient care.
- Adjustment of staffing to deal with patients with special needs.
- Strongly recommending provision of therapy at weekends.
- Sufficient staff to participate in ward rounds, case conferences and so on.

This section is followed by a range of other standards on, for example, management, patient records, equipment, policies and procedures and so on. In the section on human resources, it is stated: *"The service is directed by a rehabilitation physician"*.[76] There is no reference to any methodology for the determination of the staffing levels recommended and there is no reference to the professional bodies or any specific allied health documents on these issues.

The Indian Health Service Resources Requirements Methodology is a system designed to project the staffing needs for a specific facility or primary service area. It is available as a computer spreadsheet. The Indian Health Service is the US Department of Health and Human Services, Federal Health Programme for 'American Indians and Alaska Natives'.

The document describes what physical therapy is and lists examples of physical therapy interventions.[77] It also describes the Resources Requirement Methodology and the staffing levels formula; in essence, the level of staffing is determined by the volume of activity. Figures are given for the determination of licensed PTs and licensed PTAs. It is also stated there should be 1 WTE PT supervisor per department. Departments provide services for both out-patients and in-patients.

This is the first document internationally that we were able to locate which describes a basic methodology for the determination of physiotherapy staffing numbers for physiotherapists, assistants and clerical staffing, as well as supervisory staff.

In summary, there are very few publications on staffing level determination methodology in the international therapy literature. Also, personal contacts were unable to throw any further light on the subject, but all were very interested in this work.

For nursing, there is a reasonably substantial literature, internationally. There is also evidence that in some nursing services, there are some areas that have mandatory staffing ratios.[78]

CHAPTER 5

Are there Staffing Level Methodologies for the AHPs?

A case study

The main focus of this chapter is a case study centred on, although not exclusively about, physiotherapy staffing levels, possible methodologies and supporting information which is presented in order to exemplify the position across the AHPs.

The case study comprises a scoping exercise looking at information relating to physiotherapy and the AHPs. Although we found there was only a very small literature base about AHPs in comparison with nursing, for example, the majority of AHP publications over the last few decades related to physiotherapy. Therefore, we have used the physiotherapy case as an exemplar to illustrate the background and development of work in this area and current 'state of play' regarding methodologies for determining safe and effective staffing levels.

There's nothing new under the sun:

> "The problem is, and always has been, the lack of nationally accepted norms or guidelines from which to estimate the number of physiotherapy staff required."[79]

This was stated in a report from a meeting between the CSP and the then Department of Health and Social Security (DHSS) in May 1977, at which "*considerable interest was expressed*" in the need to establish guidance about staffing level requirements for physiotherapy services. However, the:

> "Statistical information that we required was not available. There is a paucity of recorded and validated work which would give a good, simple but flexible basic formula supplying guidance to physiotherapists and the NHS administration."[79]

Although not relevant in the healthcare provision of today, as a possible methodology for the calculation or determination of staffing levels, this report was the earliest document we could source with actual recommendations for staffing levels in physiotherapy based on a formula set up through a specific methodology. However, the document does reference 44 publications from the 1970s on various aspects of the topic which indicates a substantial level of interest in the issue at the time.

The next, and arguably most influential and significant, publications to appear on physiotherapy caseloads, case mix, workload and costing, effectiveness and measurement of efficiency in physiotherapy were the three papers emanating from the Doncaster workshops initiated and led by Joyce Williams.[3-5] The Occasional Paper No. 1 of this series, *Caseload, Casemix, Workload and Costing*,[3] was the basis for the booklet published by Williams in 1991, *Calculating Staffing Levels in Physiotherapy Services*.[2] This document broke new ground in providing a basic tool to enable physiotherapists to:
- Define and describe numerically the potential workload arising from an agreed number of cases in specified situations.
- Calculate the level of physiotherapy input available from various staffing levels.
- Describe the effect of various staffing levels in practical terms such as caseloads per staff member and input hours per bed or case.
- Assess quality and skill mix options.

The methodology did not attempt to prescribe 'norms' or ideal staffing levels, but rather to describe in practical terms the work which could be done at various levels of input. Although based on physiotherapy, the methodology was designed to be applicable to any of the AHPs. It was for managers and staff at local level to judge what was the appropriateness of the input level for the work, and for the outcomes required. The methodology used averages derived from national data surveys undertaken by Williams.

The Williams methodology[2] has been used widely in physiotherapy and other AHP services for more than 20 years and is an important point of reference; it is still used today. It has formed the basis of work in many locations throughout the UK. Clearly, it represents an important landmark in methodology for staffing level determination.

Some aspects of the Williams methodology were further developed by Jones[80] particularly in the areas of computerised information system design for AHPs for data collection, analysis and reporting for work in this area, AHP staff activity analysis, analysis of patterns of work, further data about patients and performance indicators and service costing and pricing.

The Nuffield Institute for Health Service Studies based at the University of Leeds published in 1987[81] an analysis of physiotherapist's work activities in 14 healthcare Districts in England. The study gave a comprehensive picture of physiotherapists' work activities, activity patterns in work specialties, locations and sources of casework. The methodology was robust and a wide range of information was produced. Following this a number of other groups were set up by managers around the UK to develop further workforce and staffing levels advice.

In 1988 the Wessex Regional Health Authority (RHA) Physiotherapy Working Group was established by physiotherapy managers within the Region. The purpose was to examine and report on future services and requirements,[82] to give guidelines for planning physiotherapy services over the next decade in Wessex and stimulate debate about the future shape and staffing of services. The document was prepared as:

> "A response to current national concern surrounding the supply of suitably qualified staff and the need to match demand to supply and also to the Region's service strategy ... to produce a demand forecast for the number of physiotherapy staff required."

It included an assessment of caseloads, of time typically required per case and workforce needed to provide physiotherapy services. In 1992, a substantial report written by the Institute of Manpower Studies, *Understanding Physiotherapy Staffing levels*,[83] commissioned by the Association of Chartered Physiotherapists in Management (ACPM) and the CSP was published. The content of this 63 page report includes chapters on:
- Variation in physiotherapy staffing.
- Local variation.
- Setting staffing levels.
- Measurement.
- *Recommendations for Calculating Physiotherapy Staffing for GP Referred Musculoskeletal Outpatient Services*[84] was produced by a joint working party of the CSP and ACPM in conjunction with Employment Research, and based on a survey of NHS Regions throughout the UK.

Again, this document has wide-ranging contents including a 'toolkit' to facilitate calculating physiotherapy staffing levels in GP-referred musculoskeletal outpatients.[84] The methodology section states:

> "The methodology used by many physiotherapy managers to calculate staffing levels has been based on the work of Joyce Williams. This study validates many of her recommendations and gives a sound tool from which physiotherapy managers and commissioners of physiotherapy services can accurately estimate staffing levels for new caseloads and audit current performance."

During the 1990s and early 2000s there were a number of other papers which reported work on staffing levels in detail or contribute useful background information, but these were not explicitly about the determination of staffing levels or methodologies.[85–88] During the past decade, few papers have been published relevant specifically to AHP staffing levels within the NHS. An overview includes, for example, the *'Silver Book'; Quality Care for Older People with Urgent and Emergency Care Needs*,[89] an intercollegiate document published by a number of organisations including the CSP (AGILE), The British Geriatric Society and Age UK. It discusses models of care and the multidisciplinary team approach, but there are no recommendations on staffing levels.

Some Clinical Interest Groups within the CSP have undertaken work on calculating staffing levels over recent years. AGILE, the Interest Group whose members work primarily in elderly care, produced a paper based on the research work undertaken by two of their members.[90] Again this paper is broadly based on the work of Williams.[2] In the conclusion to their research report, Squires and Hastings state:

> *"To provide a cost-effective service for older people in all care settings requires a suitable staffing profile to meet clinical standards and achieve desired results. Guidelines are given for physiotherapy staffing which can be used as a basis for negotiation in consideration of local factors and business needs. Although the model remains essentially based on professional judgement, progress has been made in that calculations are based on objective measures of quality standards, case content and venue, with audit enabling refinement and the potential for inter-provider benchmarking ... "*[90]

The Association of Chartered Physiotherapists for People with Learning Disabilities published a paper, *Calculating Physiotherapy Staffing Levels within a Service for People with Learning Disability*.[91] The aim of this paper – also based on the work of Williams[2] – was to answer a question about recommending physiotherapy staffing levels for Learning Disability services. Using part of the methodology developed by Williams, the paper concluded that an average of:

> *"... 19 patient appointments of 1 hour direct patient care per week was practicable for one WTE physiotherapist with 17 hours per week for case conferences, reviews, report writing, meetings and travel."*

The *Nottingham Demand Management Tool*[92] guidelines were researched and written by the Paediatric Physiotherapists in Management Support Group – a subgroup of the Association of Paediatric Chartered Physiotherapists. This Demand Management Tool considers the most significant factors that influence how much input any one child receives from physiotherapy, which are:
- The child's functional ability.
- The likelihood of change and the direct intervention required to achieve progress or minimise deterioration.

- The amount of indirect support required to implement and maintain the planned physiotherapy programme.
- The impact of the child changing school, nursery, etc.
- Provision of orthotics.

The tool is clinically oriented; it is a formal and *"more objective way of banding children and their needs to support the professional judgement of the physiotherapist about their priority"*. The tool was designed also to ensure equity in service provision. It is used to match the staffing hours available to the service demand and was designed to be reactive to changes in demand; it is also clinically sensitive, taking complexity into account *"rather than mere head count"*. The document was careful to make clear that it was not a 'clinical tool' as it remains up to the clinician to decide what input each child requires.

A further document, Allied Health Professionals and Healthcare Scientists Critical Care Staffing Guidance,[93] prepared on behalf of the Intensive Care Society Standards Committee National AHP and Healthcare Scientists Critical Care Advisory Group of the then Modernisation Agency (July 2003), offered guidance on physiotherapy staffing levels. In common with much other work, this lent heavily on the Williams methodology.[2] The document concluded that *"Estimation is frequently only possible and therefore a lot is based on professional judgement"*.

In addition to the documents emanating from the Clinical Interest Groups of the CSP,[90] a few documents have been published by groups in Scotland and Wales, including the AHP Capacity Calculator – User Guide.[94] This was developed by the AHP Workload Measurement and Management Project to support AHPs to:

- *"Quantify the workforce required to meet a defined workload (with/without a percentage growth) (workforce calculator).*
- *Quantify the workload a defined workforce can support (workload capacity).*
- *Develop costed Xmas tree models for a defined workforce (Christmas trees).*
- *Provide a crude efficiency quotient in the form of cost per new patient (Christmas trees)."*

This is a computerised tool that the user populates with data into the programme, the objective being that the tool quantifies workforce requirements to meet a defined workload. The calculator can be used by AHPs. The process is broken down into three steps:
1. Calculates the clinical time required to meet the current/future workload.
2. Calculates the clinical time available per WTE.
3. Calculates the number of new patients the current workforce can see per annum (pa) – quantifies the workforce required to meet the workload.

Staffing Ratio Tool (Calculating Qualified Staffing Requirements for the Physiotherapy Profession in Wales)[95] was a consensus approach tool which was produced by the All Wales Physiotherapy Managers (AWPM) Committee and issued in 2006. Before this there was:

> "... no agreed guidance document which supports physiotherapy managers in calculating qualified staffing levels across a variety of clinical specialities."

The subgroup, which was established in 2005, brought together *"physiotherapy managers from trusts across Wales who represented a range of clinical specialities"*. The purpose of the document was to provide the *"first step towards developing an agreed approach on calculating qualified physiotherapy staffing for physiotherapy services in Wales"*.

This staffing ratio tool was defined as a 'consensus approach' in which the methodology was to review the literature on staffing and other relevant documents and, where literature was not available, the AWPM subgroup proposed a:

> *"ratio based on knowledge and experience and comparing to evidence-based ratios already available. These ratios have been discussed and to a limited degree, ratified by senior clinicians across Wales as being currently appropriate."*

The document proposed three categories of cases: high complexity, intermediate and low complexity, suggesting allocation of time spent with the patient, based on the level of complexity. A wide range of staffing ratio assumptions was set out covering a large number of clinical specialties.

We contacted the Health and Social Care Information Centre;[96] there was no information available or tools on AHP staffing levels. The Health and Care Professions Council (HCPC) were also contacted to ascertain whether they have any publications, guidance or advice on staffing levels for AHP services, and they confirmed that *"HCPC does not provide guidance about staffing levels in AHP services"*.[97]

In common with much of the literature on staffing levels in the AHPs, many of the publications are now 'dated' relative to the many reforms and changes which have taken place in NHS structures, organisation, workforce and the overall political, economic, demographic and social situation. In February 2013 the Phase 3 report of the NHS Benchmarking Network on *Acute Therapies*[98] was issued to participating organisations. The project was initiated and piloted by a group of five teaching hospitals:
- Nottingham University Hospitals NHS Trust.
- Sheffield Teaching Hospitals NHS Foundation Trust.
- Leeds Teaching Hospitals NHS Trust.
- Newcastle Upon Tyne Hospitals NHS Foundation Trust.
- University Hospitals of Leicester NHS Trust.

This project covered 63 acute Trust therapy services, which employ over 7900 WTE physiotherapists and OTs. The project, which covers acute physiotherapy and OT services and looks at service models, access, activity, workforce, financial analysis, clinical outcomes and good practice, offers opportunities to develop a benchmarking approach for acute physiotherapy and occupational therapy services. There are seven objectives, one of which is to *"provide evidence for future planning, workforce design and discussions with commissioners"*. A further objective is to *"progress development of patient outcome measures"*.

There are also useful data on activity. The document includes a wealth of data and information much of which could be used in staffing level methodology determination work. It is also encouraging that one of the objectives relates to clinical outcomes and audit.

It is – of course – understandable that the data relating to individual provider organisations are made available to network participants only for comparison purposes, as they provide funding for the work. However, it is regrettable that the overarching document produced by the NHS Benchmarking Network is *"for use by network members only"*, crucially at a time when transparency, sharing and learning across the NHS are widely seen as particularly important.

Further useful data available through the NHS Electronic Staff Record[99] mechanism are available on physiotherapy workforce by Agenda for Change (AFC) grades; this can be obtained about the AHP workforce in all four countries of the UK. The information includes, for example, increases and decreases in staff by band, country specific overviews, percentage staffing changes and differences over time, data about staffing in social enterprise companies, staff headcounts and WTEs.

A paper, *Determining Hospital Workforce Requirements; A Case Study,*[100] introduces the Workload Indicators of Staffing Need (WISN) from Keele University, a method for determining staffing levels in health services. The method incorporates a form of activity analysis together with measures of *"utilisation and workload"* to determine staffing requirements. It provides a vehicle for assessing *"localised"* staffing needs that are *"believable"* and which is sharply different to historic methods. It is argued that institutional staffing norms based solely on population or size of the organisation do not adequately take into consideration these variations of need. The conceptual basis for WISN was described in 1980 and subsequently developed as an operational tool in 1984 by PJ Shipp.[101] Pilot applications of the method were undertaken in several countries including Turkey, culminating with its adoption, publication and promotion by the World Health Organization (WHO).[102]

The staffing norms in this study were all intended to be specific for the type and location of staff being considered. There are five main ways of acquiring the information:
1. Direct observation of staff activities.
2. Self-monitoring using a log or diary.
3. Questionnaires.

4. Interviewing relevant staff.
5. Expert opinion.

The results of the study in Turkey indicated:
1. Average annual working time for nurses.
2. Non-working days per year:
    i. Annual leave.
    ii. Sick leave.
    iii. Holidays.
    iv. Administrative leave.

    Total = 61 days.
    Total non-working weeks per year = 12.2 weeks.
3. Activity Standards = 39.8 weeks per year (52 weeks less 12.2 non-working weeks per year).
4. Working days = 199 days per year (39.8 weeks × 5 days per week).
5. Working hours = 1592 hours per year (199 days × 8 hours per day).

A simple model was also developed on a computer spreadsheet program to calculate the determination of standard workloads and staffing requirements for different types of services. This method echoes some aspects of the Williams methodology.[2]

In an 'Open Access' Review article, *Using Staffing Ratios for Workforce Planning; evidence on Nine Allied Health Professions*,[103] Linda Cartmill *et al.* reported the findings of their systematic literature review, which they undertook with the aim of identifying *"what workforce ratios have been used in the nine allied health professions and to identify whether these measures would be useful for planning allied health workforce requirements"*. The nine AHPs investigated through the systematic literature search were:
- Audiology.
- Dietetics and nutrition.
- Exercise physiology.
- Occupational therapy.
- Podiatry.
- Physiotherapy.
- Psychology.
- Social work.
- Speech pathology.

This comprehensive study included articles published during the period 2000–2008 inclusive. The databases examined included Medline, Cinahl, ABI/Inform, Apais Health, Business Source, Embase, Meditext, OT Seeker, Psychinfo and Pedro, and electronic searches were also undertaken of Australian

Health Review, Cochrane Library Economic Evaluation Database, website of Public Health Research Unit for the UK NHS and the Service Delivery and Organisation Programme of the National Institute for Health Research. Requests were also made to the professional bodies of the nine professions in Australia for any available documentation on workplace ratios. Their websites were also checked for any published information. Some 1207 papers were identified and were screened by title and abstract for compliance with the inclusion and exclusion criteria. A total of 989 papers were excluded. Following a second detailed review and application of inclusion and exclusion criteria only 30 relevant articles were identified and in 12 figures were given for the ratio of *"different AHPs to bed or patient numbers"*. Of these, only one scored highly on study quality criteria.

The study[103] concluded:

> *"Use of staffing ratios to determine appropriate staff numbers can be a useful tool to guide service planning and delivery. This tool has been successfully used in nursing particularly in the acute care setting. This review aimed to find out if allied health workforce ratios existed and if these ratios could be used in allied health service planning. However, there were few examples of staffing ratios found for AHPs and only one of these was a staffing ratio linked to clinical outcomes ...*
>
> *It is not possible from the evidence presented to use workforce ratios to plan for allied health requirements in general settings such as a general hospital or a community setting."*

In their conclusion the authors state:

> *"As the population ages and the incidence of chronic disease rises there will be increased demand for allied health services. Health managers and policy makers will need access to appropriate evidence based research to guide workforce planning to best meet community health needs."*

The review authors found that:

> *"Research on staffing ratios for allied health practitioners is scarce and lags behind nursing and medicine. There is little available on allied health requirements in general hospital settings such as orthopaedics and surgery and also in general community settings ..."*

This comprehensive study[103] provides further evidence in support of our own view that there is no generally accepted methodology in place for the determination of safe and effective staffing levels in AHP services, and that on the rare occasions when evidence can be found for staffing ratios, these do not relate to identified need, the many elements of demand, dependency, quality requirements, desired outcomes and so on. Safe and effective staffing must be based on all of these and other factors to enable staffing levels to be matched to the many parameters of demand.

CHAPTER 6

Methodology for Determining Safe and Effective Staffing Levels for the AHPs – The Jones/Jenkins Approach

Introduction

As the previous chapters in this book demonstrate there are many reasons why urgent work needs to be done on the development of a transparent, accurate, relevant and robust methodology, which is valid and reliable for determining safe and effective staffing levels for the AHPs within the NHS, and other healthcare providers. There is also a requirement from within the AHPs themselves, both nationally and internationally, to have sound data available for business cases, service improvement and innovation, redesign, maintenance of current services or implementing change, and for managing services effectively on a day-to-day basis.

Much of the data and information are already there within the services to enable the introduction of a rigorous evidence-based approach to staffing level determination. The 'trick' is to pull the required data and information together to enable the relevant calculations to be made. Implementation of our methodology will enable this and will be to the benefit of the patients we serve, resulting in safe, effective and efficient service provision, as well as of benefit to the employer organisations, staff, commissioners, planners and others.

In this chapter, we set out our methodology for determining safe and effective staffing levels together with tools, techniques and calculation examples that we have developed, tried, tested and used in our own management and leadership practice over many years. The methodology also draws on our experience as managers, leaders and clinicians, and on our work in healthcare research and consultancy. It incorporates approaches and elements of methodologies and the ideas of others such as those of Williams,[2] which we have adapted for use in AHP healthcare provision today.

What it's not

Our approach does not attempt to lay down or prescribe specific staffing levels or norms for staffing levels. There are no recommendations, for example, on numbers of WTE staff per size of population such as: 'N' number of staff per 100,000 population in the catchment area, or 'N' HCPC registered or assistants staff per number of admitted patients, or the ratio of HCPC registered staff to non-HCPC registered assistants and so on. Rather, it is about using the data and information we already have within our services and organisations, together with any benchmarking data we can obtain, to make the relevant calculations.

What is our main aim?

Our main aim is to show how safe and effective staffing levels can be calculated using the data and information already available in most services.

The four countries of the UK

As indicated in previous chapters various approaches to staffing level determination have been pursued in the four countries of the UK. However, there is no reason why our methodology should not be used across the UK as a whole, as it is applicable to any service in possession of the necessary data. To use the same methodology across the board would be economical in use of time, save money and enable benchmarking exercises to be undertaken across boundaries as appropriate. We hope this approach might also be of interest internationally, and perhaps could be used in some other countries. Many AHP delegates attending masterclasses we have run overseas have kindly indicated their interest and enthusiasm and have asked us to keep them updated on the development work.

Basis of our methodology, the concept – what you do

The concepts underpinning our methodology are: firstly, a full assessment of the work required to provide the new service, for the service redesign or the work requirements in an existing service which is under review; this represents the *demand*. The next process is calculation and analysis of the 'average' annual activity/workload capacity which can be undertaken safely and effectively by an 'average' WTE staff member (by grade/band and AHP) working in a specific clinical situation or specialty and then aggregating this figure by the number of staff required to match the projected annual workload for the ward, section, department, specialty or specific service to be staffed; the *capacity*. The result of the aggregation process provides data on the projected potential activity or workload capacity of a given number of staff. In any given clinical situation the balance of the skill mix of the staff providing the service is crucial, in order that the correct levels of expertise and experience, from most experienced 'high level' clinicians to the most junior or newly qualified member of the team, are available to achieve the best outcomes possible. The expertise and experience required is dependent upon the particular patient cohort need, taking account of, for example, clinical complexity, dependency, local circumstances, acute or chronic conditions and so on. Therefore, calculations must take into account the grade mix required within the team.

We stated in Chapter 1 of this book that an analysis of the elements required to provide quality services would not be included here, as this is a vast and complex topic in its own right and needs to be discussed in depth. However, it is essential that we emphasise the overriding importance of quality service provision in relation to the methodology. It is not simply a question of considering the demand as a purely statistical entity; it is essential that a full understanding of quality issues in the widest sense is incorporated. This should not be a purely mechanistic process; sufficient time must be incorporated to enable patient care to be carried out with compassion, respecting dignity and taking into account the individual needs of patients. The role of AHP managers and leaders is crucial in clearly 'flagging' this up, as proper advice and input on relevant skill mix, levels of expertise and experience must be considered. It is also essential that thinking around this incorporates staff development, the need for R&D, training needs and many other parameters. *Demand* must include reference to these and many other quality factors and the *capacity* then designed to match.

The steps for calculation

Step 1	What specialty (patient cohort) is the service to be provided for?
Step 2	Consider the dependency level of patients within the patient cohort for whom the service is to be provided.
Step 3	What is the projected annual caseload and throughput – annual workload, (demand) – for the proposed new service, redesigned service or for an existing service which is under review?
Step 4	Include the quality parameters required to ensure safe and effective care.
Step 5	Assess which AHP services are required.
Step 6	Assess what levels of expertise and experience are needed from each AHP group, balance of skill mix (grade/banding of staff required) for the specific patient cohort.
Step 7	Calculate the 'average' annual activity/workload capacity which can be undertaken by an 'average' WTE staff member (by grade/band and AHP profession) required to work in the specific specialty or service area.
Step 8	Total the required individual WTEs annual caseload capacities to give the overall annual caseload capacity.
Step 9	Ensure that overall staffing capacity matches the anticipated annual workload identified in Step 3 (above) for each of the AHP services required.
Step 10	Calculate staffing costs from the number of staff in each grade/band (skill mix required) for the team.

The essence of the methodology is to ensure that the annual staff workload capacity matches the identified annual caseload of the proposed new service, redesigned service or existing service under discussion.

It is important to note that the staffing requirement will be different for each of the AHP professions included in the team for each specific service, as the work of each AHP professional group differs greatly and the time required for a given patient throughput varies according to the patient needs and dependency within specific specialty areas. A mistake sometimes made by non-AHP colleagues involved in this work is that all the AHPs are taken to be the same. However, the 16 professions included in the HCPC remit (*see* Appendix 1) have greatly differing inputs in different specialty areas. For example, in diabetology, dietetics and podiatry may be substantially involved as service providers, but there will be different volumes of input between these two, while speech and language therapy is not generally required. The steps in the process are set out in the box on the previous page.

A simple calculation, for example, might be: if the throughput of a particular service is 3000 patients pa and an individual WTE can treat 600 new patients pa, then approximately 5 WTE staff will be required for that workload. (3000/600 = 5 staff) in a unidisciplinary situation.

However, it is not quite that simple as different staff grades will be able to treat different numbers of patients depending on experience, expertise, other duties and so on; therefore, the calculation for a team providing a service for 3000 patients will need to be flexed to reflect the different workload capacities of the various grades in the skill mix required. A further important factor that must be considered is the mix of AHPs required. Therefore, the most straightforward method is to consider each AHP group separately. For example, in the case of stroke patient care, consider requirements for physiotherapy, OT and speech and language therapy separately, as these provide different elements of the care required by this patient cohort. We have found that more often than not the methodology works best where it is applied to each AHP group required for the service. It must also be borne in mind that a caseload of 600 patients doesn't mean just 600 interventions (face-to-face patient contacts) in the year, as each patient may, for the purposes of this example, need an average of three follow-up face-to-face treatment interventions, i.e. 600 patients × 4 treatments each on average, equals 2400 contacts per WTE. This shows that new patient throughput pa does not equal the entire workload by a long way, as many of the patients will receive a number of treatment interventions during their episode of care.

The AHP working week in the UK

Under the Agenda for Change regulations in the UK, the working week for AHPs is 37.5 hours per week. Using this figure the number of hours available for work pa can be calculated. Our research shows that on average a WTE AHP member of staff works for 41 weeks pa. This takes account of:
- Annual leave of up to 33 days pa.
- 8 bank holidays.

- Average study leave pa.
- Average sickness leave pa.
- Other authorised absence pa.

The calculation for working hours available pa is:

    37.5 hours per week × 41 weeks = 1537.5 available working hours pa.

However, this does not mean that clinical staff are working in face-to-face direct patient contact all of that time as there is a wide range of necessary and legitimate activities which constitute the full working role in all clinical posts.

Workload data examples

The 'snapshot' of data set out here is not intended to provide 'norms', mandatory staffing levels or recommended figures; calculations must be undertaken on a local basis using the most reliable, valid and robust information available at the time. Examples 1–3 (below) are related to one another and demonstrate how capacity can be calculated. Our methodology is applicable to all clinical areas using the relevant average time per face-to-face contact and other relevant data.

Example 1 – A typical AHP
- 1 WTE = 41 working weeks/pa = 1537.5 hours.
- An average annual caseload for a Band 6 might be 511 new patients pa = 12.5 new patients (np) per week. (511 nps/41 weeks = 12.46 np).
- Appointment times = 30 minutes.
- Average contacts per patient = 5 (a first appointment and 4 follow-ups) = 2.5 hours each episode.
- 511 patients × 2.5 hours = 1277.5 hours patient activity pa.
- Leaving 260 hours for 'other' activity (1537.5 – 1277.5) = 6.5 hours per week per WTE.

Example 2 – A service department with 10 WTE
- Number of staff = 10 WTE.
- 15,375 hours work available capacity in the department (10 WTE × 1537.5 hours).
- Capacity 5110 np pa (using an average 511 np pa per WTE × 10 staff).
- 12,775 hours pa patient contact work (5110 × 2.5 hours).
- 2600 hours available for 'other' activity (15375 – 12775 hours).

> Example 3 – A worked capacity example
> - Total annual referrals to department of 10 staff = 5610 average pa.
> - Waiting list = 500 patients = 1250 hours work (500 patients × 5 treatments × 30 min = 1250 hours).
> - Need 1 WTE more activity to meet this demand.

We have discussed our methodology with colleagues in several countries where the working week and other parameters are different from those in the UK. Colleagues in NZ provided the figures on which the next two examples are presented; these turn out to be rounded figures which we believe helps clarify the methodology further:

> Example 4 – an example from NZ
> - 45 working weeks per year per 1 WTE.
> - 40 hours per working week per WTE.
> - 40 × 45 = 1800 hours pa per WTE capacity.
> - 25% non-patient activity = 10 hours per week.
> - 30 hours per WTE patient contact per week = 1350 patient contact hours pa.
> - Average patient contact time = 1.5 hours per patient episode.
> - 900 new patient pa capacity = 20 np per week per WTE.
> - 1 WTE for 45 weeks = 1350 hours pa (30 × 45).
> - 10 hours per week for other activity = 450 hours pa per WTE.

> Example 5 – an NZ Service with 10 WTE
> - 10 WTE members of staff.
> - = 18,000 hours per Department pa, i.e. 45 weeks × 40 hours per week × 10 WTE.
> - = 9000 new patients capacity pa.
> - = 13,500 hours patient contact (1.5 hours × 9000).
> - = 4500 hours for other activity pa.

The principal method for calculation used in all five examples set out here is applicable to all AHP services in all clinical areas. The essential point is that data from within the service or benchmarking exercises are used. Average caseloads can be calculated from service statistical returns on numbers of WTE staff in particular areas, new patients pa, follow-ups and throughputs pa, for example. It is also important to understand the percentage face-to-face contact time and patient-related activity relative to non-patient-related activity. It is important to keep in mind that the non-patient-related activity is also legitimate and important work, contributing to the overall service quality. Our research over many years indicates that the figure is usually 70–80% for patient-related activity for the most clinically deployed staff grades, while the percentages are likely to be less for categories of staff with other commitments such as management roles.

In a national survey of physiotherapy activity[104] which we undertook in 2011, the average number of new patients referred to musculoskeletal out-patient physiotherapy departments from 69 organisations was 11,668 pa. The minimum number of patient treatment contacts per episode of care reported was 1 and the maximum 5.9. The average number of contacts per episode of care was 3.31 which gave a first to follow-up ratio of 1:2.31. With regard to the number of new patients treated *each week* by different grade/band of WTE physiotherapy staff, the figures provided by 14 services were:

- Band 5   11.55 np.
- Band 6   13.21 np.
- Band 7   12.54 np.
- Band 8a   12.07 np.

Our survey of data provided for 2009–10[105] indicated average caseloads per WTE in physiotherapy musculoskeletal out-patient services of:
- Band 5   2078 face-to-face contacts.
- Band 6   2227 face-to-face contacts.
- Band 7   2237 face-to-face contacts.
- Band 8a   2000 face-to-face contacts.

For trauma and orthopaedic in-patient physiotherapy services the average face-to-face treatment contacts per patient in 21 services was 4.8, while in physiotherapy services for acute hospital in-patient wards for patients with stroke the average number of contacts per patient was 10.3.[104]

Most AHP services will have or be able to obtain the 'raw material' for undertaking these types of calculations locally using their own throughput, caseload, staffing and other data. Some will have access to benchmarking data[98] and others may be able to work with colleagues to create their own benchmarks.

Setting staffing levels needs to be done on the basis of agreed workloads for the specific service or part of service, section, department and so on. Here the staffing level needed for the agreed workload is calculated. We recommend this method as it is in keeping with business practice for service contracts, service level agreements, and it is patient and service driven rather than staff based.

Agreeing the staffing level needed on the basis of the agreed or projected caseload is a tried and tested methodology which is straightforward, easy to use and is based on evidence.

We have developed several tools and processes to support our work in this and parallel areas such as demand and capacity management, benchmarking development and so on. Some of these tools we have used for many years and some have also been used by others working on staffing level determination, and we set out an overview of some of these (below). It is certainly true that there can be a number of solutions to specific problems, but we believe that the guidance we offer will assist the determination of staffing levels based on a logical process. There are a number of important factors which will support an appreciation of the 'big picture' in staffing level work.

We have extracted and edited part of a chapter from one of our previous books which discusses our activity sampling system in detail, together with demonstrating how the data can be collected; we also provide the pro forma for the data collection exercises with notes on how this can be done. This, and the section on benchmarking which follows later in this chapter, are both reproduced by permission of Radcliffe Publishing Ltd, for which we thank them.

Staff activity analysis

AHP managers and leaders need an accurate picture of workforce activity for staffing level determination, throughput, what work is undertaken, who does it, where it happens, what sort of service or interventions are provided and so on. A thorough understanding of work activity is essential to service and workforce planning, development of staffing profiles for specific programmes and for a wide range of other purposes, such as for costing and pricing, evidence-based staff deployment, capacity and demand management, implementation of 7-day-a-week service provision and staff activity analysis. Such information also facilitates evidence-based service development and strategy, enabling critical evaluation of different staff activities to support specific projects.

Our activity analysis technique is helpful in understanding management and administrative inputs and supporting analysis of patterns of work for capacity and demand management. If carried out in collaboration with colleagues from other organisations, the approach can also be used for benchmarking exercises. Activity analysis is also important in monitoring and supporting a range of clinical governance parameters. It is a method of sampling volumes and types of activity undertaken by AHP staff in all grades and specialties on a regular 'snapshot' basis, using a sample activity data collection process based on a template form. Data can then be extracted for use in a programme for reporting and subsequent analysis and interpretation. The different components of patient-related work and non-patient care work need to be understood for effective and efficient service provision and management in the increasingly business oriented environment.

This approach has been used in our services over many years and the data obtained used for management and clinical purposes and for benchmarking between locations, as well as in service reviews we have undertaken.

ACTIVITY PROFORMA

PROFESSIONAL GROUP: _____

DATE	SITE	LOCATION	CLINICIAN CODE	BAND	YOUR POST NAME/ROTATION	ABSENT? REASON

ACTIVITY		HOURS	MINS
PATIENT RELATED			
FACE-TO-FACE CONTACT (Individual)			
FACE-TO-FACE CONTACTS (Group)			
TELEPHONE CONTACTS with patient or relative			
WARD ROUNDS			
CASE CONFERENCES			
LIAISON WITH OTHER SERVICES – related to patient care			
ADMINISTRATION – patient related			
HOME ASSESSMENT VISITS			
CLINICS			
OTHER (patient related)			
NON-PATIENT RELATED			
LIAISON WITH OTHER SERVICES – not related to patient			
ADMINISTRATION – not patient related			
MANAGEMENT DUTIES			
STUDY LEAVE			
TRAVEL			
STAFF/TEAM MEETINGS			
IN-SERVICE TRAINING/EDUCATION			
TEACHING/TRAINING	Your professional group		
TEACHING/TRAINING	Students		
TEACHING/TRAINING	Other		
CLINICAL SUPERVISION			
OTHER (non-patient related)			
Your contracted working hours Today			
No. of group sessions you have done Today			
No. of patients on your caseload Today			

FIGURE 1 AHP services activity sample pro forma

Tips for implementation
- Ensure the data collection form is fully tested and piloted in your service.
- Involve all team members. Explain the purpose and importance of the exercise.
- Computer support and analysis is essential.
- Forward planning for the sample enquiry is important.
- Thorough teaching of definitions of the data items is essential.
- It is essential to share results and outcomes with all teams taking part in the sample.

AHP services activity sample pro forma: briefing notes
Understanding staff activity and the way we spend our working hours is important for management, clinical, and financial purposes and when developing new services and redesigning current ones. The activity sample can be run as a 'snapshot', for example, a week several times during the year, a month or two, or for a more comprehensive analysis, a 13-week quarter can be used, doing it on 1 (differing) day per week, that is, week 1 Monday, week 2 Tuesday and so on. A consistent approach to completing the form is needed, so these briefing notes should be shared with all staff who are to undertake the survey. The form is divided into four main sections:
1. General information.
2. Patient-related activity.
3. Non-patient-related activity.
4. Contracted working hours and caseloads.
    - Each member of staff completes a new form on each day of the activity sample whether working that day or not.
    - The main activity sample takes place Monday to Friday inclusive, but members of staff working at the weekend will also be requested to complete forms for those days.
    - The form should be completed by HCPC Registered staff and non-registered assistants.

The Form Part 1 – General information
Professional group: The AHP professional group of which you are a member (including assistants), e.g. occupational therapy, dietetics, physiotherapy, etc.

Date: The date on which the form is completed. Forms must be completed on the same day as the activity takes place. It is best to do this as you go through the day to be sure of accuracy.

Site: This is where you are working, e.g. District General Hospital, community hospital, domiciliary, or special school. If you work in more than one site on one day, a new form should be completed for each site.

Location: The place within your organisation where the interventions take place, e.g. wards, physiotherapy department, podiatry clinics, patients' homes.

Clinician code: The individual staff code (whatever is used within the organisation for your personal identifier).

Band: Agenda for Change grade.

Your post name/rotation: e.g. clinical specialist in ... Band 5 in-patient rotation, out-patient department assistant.

Absent? Reason: Why you are not working today, e.g. annual leave, part-time do not work today, study leave, sickness, etc.

The Form Part 2 – Patient-related activity

Enter hours and minutes spent on each activity accurately:
- Face-to-face contact with individual patients.
- Face-to-face contact with patients in groups.
- Telephone contacts with patients, relatives and carers.
- Ward rounds.
- Case conferences.
- Liaison with other services related to patient care.
- Administrative work related to patient care, e.g. record-keeping.
- Home assessment visits with or without the patient in attendance.
- Clinics.
- Other patient-related activity to capture others not included above (must be strictly patient-related).

The Form Part 3 – Non-patient-related activity

Enter hours and minutes spent on each activity accurately:
- Liaison with other services, not related to patient care; could be for a wide range of reasons.
- Administration; not patient-related, e.g. sending out appointments.
- Management duties: all work involved in service management or management duties within the organisation.
- Study leave – you are on study leave yourself.
- Travel: in the community, between sites or locations, walking the corridors.
- Staff and team meetings.
- In-service education/training: attendance (not leading or presenting).
- Teaching and training: when you are leading, presenting or giving this for:
    —your own professional group.
    —students.
    —others.
- Clinical supervision: providing or attending.
- Other non-patient-related activities not captured above.

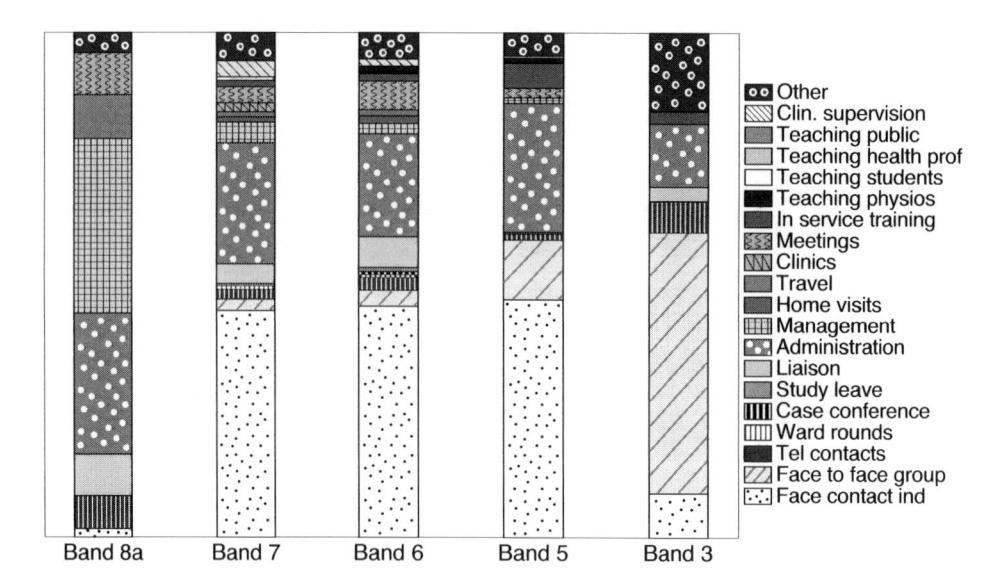

54 SAFE AND EFFECTIVE STAFFING LEVELS FOR THE ALLIED HEALTH PROFESSIONS

FIGURE 2 Subdivision of staff time by staff band.

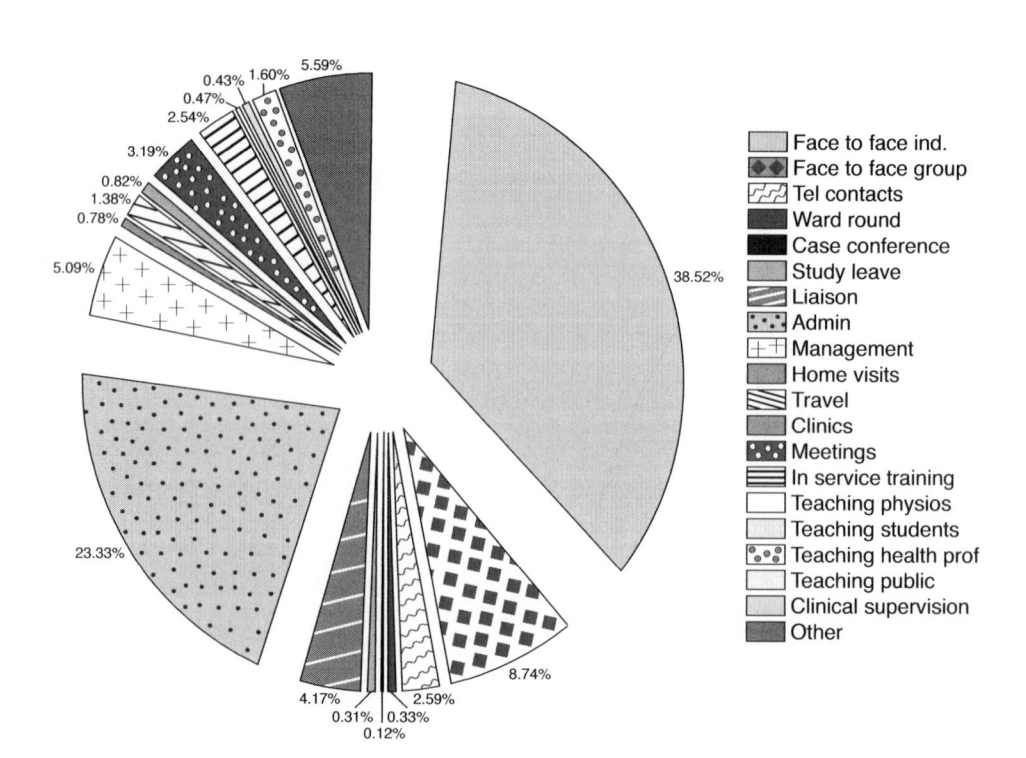

FIGURE 3 Subdivision of staff time; all staff.

The Form Part 4 – About your contracted hours and caseload

Your contracted working hours today: the number of hours you are contracted to work that day; if part time and not working that day, indicate this.

Number of group sessions you have done today.

Number of patients on your caseload today: how many patients did you see or should you have seen, including 'DNAs' or 'unable to attends' (UTA).

Example of reports from activity sample data

The activity sample data can be analysed and the results shown in tabular or graphical formats as shown in Figures 2–4. This is the aggregated activity for both patient-related and non-patient-related activity. These can be broken down to look at any specific parameter and make comparisons with any of the others. This type of analysis is an important and powerful tool and needs to be used in association with qualitative measures. By understanding the way that staff spend their time and the division between patient contact time and non-patient contact time, the manager is able to workforce plan effectively to ensure efficient staffing. The data also contribute to the determination of safe and effective staffing levels.

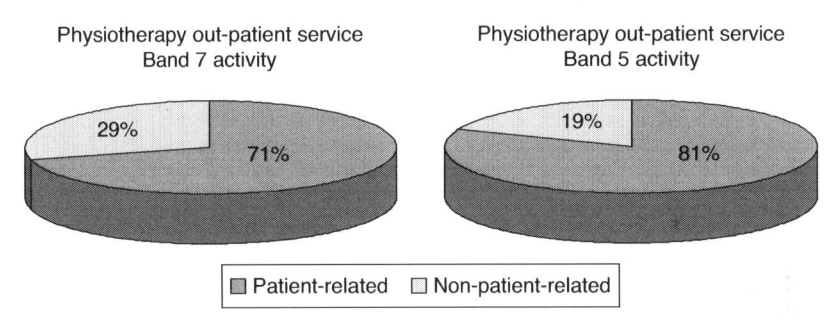

FIGURE 4 Comparison of out-patient staff: patient-related to non-patient-related activity by Band 7 and Band 5, physiotherapy out-patient service.

Data and information management

Information management is an essential aspect of AHP management. Information management and technology (IM&T) offers many benefits to AHP managers, clinicians, and service users, including the following:
- To support the determination of safe and effective staffing levels.
- Support to strategic and operational management.
- Support to good business and staff management.
- Identification of trends.
- Warning of potential adverse events.
- More effective and efficient record-keeping.
- Better management of patient care.

- Development of and access to the evidence base.
- Audit, research and development.
- Use in many aspects of clinical governance reporting.
- Use in human resource management.

Whether the service is in primary, secondary or tertiary care, voluntary, private or other sectors, management of the service directly impacts on the quality of care provided. IM&T are essential tools to support all elements of quality management to enable service effectiveness and efficiency, management of change, and service redesign. The effective use of data to manage services enables AHP managers and leaders to contribute fully.

Application of activity sampling in the context of staffing level determination

This system of activity sampling and analysis was originally developed 30 years ago. The activity data collection pro forma was piloted and prototyped with substantial staff input and comment and tested across 15 organisations. Since that time we have used and further developed the process with staff input at all levels.

Average levels of patient-related activity

This method generally indicates an across AHP patient-related activity percentage time use in the region of 70–80%. This accords with work undertaken by Williams[2] and the Nuffield Institute.[81] The sampling work we have undertaken, both in our own services and in service reviews, also indicates consistent levels within these parameters for AHP patient-related activity, with some variation between different AHP professions and grades/bands. The proportion of patient-related and non-patient-related activity is important in the calculation of safe and effective staffing levels. Although clinical staff are employed to provide a clinical service, it must be recognised that there are non-patient-related activities which are crucial to the provision of effective and efficient services and that these activities are essential elements in the job content of AHP clinicians.

Benchmarking AHP services

Benchmarking is an invaluable means of enhancing understanding of your service's performance, achieved through making comparisons with other organisations. It demonstrates how your service is performing in relation to similar AHP services and will also indicate whether the full potential of the workforce and other resources is being fully realised. If, as AHP managers and leaders, we have no idea what the standards are for a wide range of parameters, we cannot compare, to establish the relationship between our organisation and others. Benchmarking can be an invaluable tool in safe and effective staffing level determination and is also often used as part of service review and for quality improvement initiatives. The technique is a widely used management tool that had its origins in the manufacturing industry and is now used in public services, including healthcare.

Introducing our Benchmarking Tool

We have developed this AHP benchmarking tool,[106,107] which can be used by managers to help set standards and monitor whether or not these are being met in terms of workforce, resources, activity, availability, access and so on. To date, there has been no universally accepted 'validated tool' or process available to AHP managers and their teams to use and undertake this work. In view of this and as a result of our own experience in undertaking service reviews evaluation and consultancy, we recognised that a basic benchmarking process, which is evidence-based, would be helpful to AHP managers and wider healthcare organisations.

Initially the tool included a wide range of specialties, but following piloting and advice received from heads of AHP services and clinicians, we decreased the number of categories included to facilitate ease of completion and opportunity for comparisons to be made. Our benchmarking tool is designed to be objective and a straightforward process, which can either be used to review your own service in isolation, or to make comparisons with aspects of other services, or with other services in their entirety. We hope the tool will support and be helpful to AHP managers undertaking benchmarking exercises.

How to use the tool – briefing notes

The tool has five sections:
1. Your organisation.
2. Your professional group.
3. In-patient services.
4. Out-patient services.
5. Community services.

The purpose of these briefing notes is to ensure – as far as possible – a consistent and accurate methodology for collecting the data between the provider services participating in benchmarking exercises. Organisations taking part may be widely dispersed across the region, country, or between countries, and there are differing practices and definitions in use in different places. Therefore, uniformity of approach will help to ensure that the data collected enables valid comparisons and consistent interpretation.

It is possible to select only a few categories for benchmarking or to include the whole service. The more generic categories that are chosen to describe the service, the more likely it will be to find a comparator to benchmark with. Therefore, consider very carefully the categories you select to benchmark. We recognise, for example, that some areas have elderly care wards and in other areas, elderly care is part of general medicine; we have amalgamated these and have one category, general medicine.

We also recognise that different professions have different subspecialisms; for example, gastroenterology is likely to be a high input for dietitians, but physiotherapists may include this in-patient activity as part of general medicine.

The data collection spreadsheet is divided into five sections.

Section 1. Your Organisation – General Information

Only one Section 1 form needs filling in per organisation.
- Date: the date the form is completed.
- Provider name: the name of your organisation.
- Professional groups being benchmarked: please list the professions for benchmarking and then insert the WTE HCPC registered staff, WTE non-registered clinical staff, WTE admin and clerical, total WTE all staff.
- Contact details for the person completing the form: generally the most senior AHP manager in the service. Give name and email contact.
- Provider type: e.g. Acute Trust, Community Services, Care Trust, Foundation Trust, Tertiary Provider, Integrated Health Board, etc.
- Catchment population for your organisation: state the population in thousands.
- Total number of beds in the organisation: list the current declared bed stock.
- Budget for services being benchmarked: first list the services being benchmarked, then include the total budget, pay budget, and non-pay budget for all of the professional groups combined and finally add up the columns to give the grand totals.
- Indicate whether you want your organisation's name to be kept anonymous: highlight Yes or No.

Each individual profession will need to complete sections 2–5 inclusive as appropriate.

| **BENCHMARKING AHP SERVICES** |
| **1. Your Organisation** |

Professional groups being benchmarked (list):
1
2
3
4
5
6

Contact details for the person completing the form (optional)
Name:
Position:
Email address:

Provider Type (please tick):
1. Acute Trust
2. Foundation Trust:
3. Care Trust
4. PCT Provider
5. Mental Health Trust
6. Combined Acute and Community
7. Tertiary
8. Other (please specify):

Catchment Population:
Total number of beds in organisation:

Budget for services being benchmarked (list professional groups)			
1. Physio	Total Budget = £	Pay Budget = £	Non-Pay Budget = £
2. OT	Total Budget = £	Pay Budget = £	Non-Pay Budget = £
3. SALT	Total Budget = £	Pay Budget = £	Non-Pay Budget = £
4. Dietetics	Total Budget = £	Pay Budget = £	Non-Pay Budget = £
5. Podiatry	Total Budget = £	Pay Budget = £	Non-Pay Budget = £
6. Other			
Grand Totals:	£	£	£

Do you want to keep your organisation's name anonymous? (Please identify) Y/N

TABLE 1 Your Organisation

Section 2. Professional group and staffing
- Total WTE managerial staff: fill in the boxes that are not shaded as appropriate. For staff with mixed managerial and clinical roles, include here the approximate WTE of their time assigned to management duties.
- Total WTE clinical staff for your professional group (excluding consultants): this includes every member of staff you employ, working within your organisation.
- Total WTE AHP consultants.
- Total WTE assistant and support staff.
- Total WTE administration and clerical staff.
- Staff from your professional group you provide to other organisations: this would include the staff that you employ and that you may have service-level agreements to provide to another organisation, e.g. rotational staff, hospices, etc.
- Total staff: add up the rows to give your total staff by band for the staff group.

2. Your Professional Group and Staffing

The Name of Your Professional Group:

	WTE Registered Staff										WTE Non-Registered Staff				
	Band 5	Band 6	Band 7	Band 8a	Band 8b	Band 8c	Band 8d	Band 9	Director		Band 2	Band 3	Band 4	Band 5	Band 6
Total WTE Managerial Staff															
Total WTE Clerical staff															
Total WTE Clinical Staff for your professional group															
Staff from your professional group you provide to other organisations															

TABLE 2 Professional group and staffing

Section 3. In-patient services

An in-patient service is defined as:

> One where patients (clients) occupy beds overnight as part of their episode of care. This may be in acute or community settings and in health or social care.

The list of specialities is not exhaustive, but it is hoped that most therapy services will be able to group their total in-patient activity under several of the categories listed. It is not intended for every specialty to be used by every professional group. Where highly specialist or tertiary services are provided, please list them in the 'other' category – though this may make it more difficult to benchmark.

- Your professional group: name the professional group you are reporting information for.
- Beds per specialty: for the specialties you are providing data for; indicate the current number of beds in the unshaded boxes.
- WTE registered staff, i.e. staff registered with the HCPC.
- WTE non-registered staff, i.e. assistants and clinical support staff; do not include clerical staff in this section.
- Total staff: add up the rows to give your total staff for the specialty.
- New patients last year: total number of new patients for the last financial year.
- Total contacts last year: total face-to-face contacts for the last financial year.
- 7-day service yes/no: this includes routine working, even if only for part of the day and not an 'on-call' service which can be audited separately.
- Validated clinical outcome measures used: identify at the bottom of the sheet the names of the validated outcome measures used.
- Clinical specialties: for each of these broadly defined clinical specialties, enter the relevant data in each column. Some clinical specialties listed will not require detailed benchmark scrutiny for every professional group, e.g. gastroenterology is likely to be pertinent to dietetic services, whereas physiotherapy may group this service as part of general medical services. Similarly, it is unlikely that podiatry services will input to ITU regularly. It is anticipated that data will be provided for a wide range of specialties for each profession.
- Other (please specify): if your in-patient service is very different from one in the list, e.g. tertiary service, cardiothoracic or neurosurgery, identify it and provide data.
- Day surgery: provide data for therapy input to day surgery services, i.e. where there is no overnight stay.
- Total staff: add up columns to give your total staff by band.

3. In-patient Services

Name of Your Professional Group:

Clinical Specialties	Beds per specialty	WTE Registered Staff									WTE Non-Registered Staff				WTE total staff	New patients last year	Total contacts last year	Average length of stay	Validated clinical outcome measures used? Yes/No
		Band 5	Band 6	Band 7	Band 8a	Band 8b	Band 8c	Band 8d	Band 9	Band 2	Band 3	Band 4	Band 5					
Community Hospital Rehabilitation Ward																		
Elderly Care																		
General Medicine																		
General Surgery																		
ITU																		
Medical Assessment Unit/Emergency Admissions Unit																		
Head and Neck																		
Oncology																		
Paediatrics																		
Stroke Unit – acute																		
Stroke Unit – rehab																		
Neurology (not stroke)																		

TABLE 3 In-patient services

Section 4. Out-patient services

An out-patient is someone who attends a hospital or clinic for treatment that does not require an overnight stay.

This section is to gather information on patients who meet this definition. This could include both adult and children's services and may be in primary or secondary care, normally in a healthcare setting. The list of specialities is not exhaustive, and is intended to give a reasonable level of specialisation for each profession, but also recognises that to list every therapy subspecialty would be an exhaustive process. It is not intended for every specialty to be used by every professional group. Where highly specialist or tertiary services are provided, please list them in the 'other' category; this may make it more difficult to benchmark, so only use when really necessary.

- Your professional group: name the professional group you are reporting information for.
- WTE registered staff, i.e. staff registered with the HCPC.
- WTE non-registered staff, i.e. assistants and clinical support staff (do not include clerical staff in this section).
- Total staff: add up rows to give your total staff for the specialty.
- Group treatment: answer yes or no for each specialty.
- Average number of new patients/week per WTE: where staff are set a target number of new patients per week, please enter this number for each specialty that this applies to.
- New patients last year: total number of new patients for the last financial year.
- Total contacts last year: total face-to-face contacts for the last financial year.
- DNA per cent: this includes all DNA and UTA for first and follow-up appointments as a percentage of all appointments.
- Validated clinical outcome measures used: identify at the bottom of the sheet the names of the validated outcome measures used.
- Out-patient specialties: for each of these broadly defined specialties, enter the relevant data in each column. Some specialties listed will not be relevant to all professional groups, e.g. dysfluency is likely to be only a speech and language therapy specialty, whereas wheelchair and seating clinics may be pertinent for both physiotherapy and occupational therapy. It is anticipated that data will be provided for a wide range of specialties for each profession, but not each and every one.
- Other (please specify): if your out-patient service is different from one in the list, please identify it and provide data; this may make it more difficult to benchmark, so only use when really necessary.

4. Out-patient Services

Name of Your Professional Group:

	WTE Registered Staff								WTE Non-Registered Staff				Average no. new patients/ week per WTE	New patients last year	Total contacts last year	DNA %	1st: Follow-up ratio	Validated clinical outcome measures used? Yes/No
	Band 5	Band 6	Band 7	Band 8a	Band 8b	Band 8c	Band 8d	Band 9	Band 2	Band 3	Band 4	Band 5						
Cardiac Rehab																		
Communication																		
Diabetes																		
Dysfluency (SALT)																		
Fracture Clinic																		
Gastroenterology																		
Group Activities																		
Hand Therapy																		
Head and Neck																		
Hydrotherapy																		
Musculoskeletal																		
Neurology (excluding stroke)																		
Occupational Health																		
Paediatrics																		
Pain Management																		
Palliative Care																		
Pulmonary Rehab																		
Rheumatology																		
Stroke																		
Voice (SALT)																		
Women's/Men's Health																		

TABLE 4 Out-patient services

Section 5. Community services

Community services are those AHP services that are provided away from hospital premises and are neither in-patient services nor out-patient. Examples would include services provided to education and a range of community-based facilities such as GP surgeries, community clinics and children's centres.

- Your professional group: name the professional group you are reporting information for.
- WTE registered staff, i.e. staff registered with the HCPC.
- WTE non-registered staff, i.e. assistants and clinical support staff (do not include clerical staff in this section).
- Total staff: add up rows to give your total staff for the specialty.
- Group treatment: answer yes or no for each specialty.
- New patients last year: total number of new patients for the last financial year.
- Total contacts last year: total face-to-face contacts for the last financial year.
- 7-day service yes/no: this includes routine working, even if only for part of the day and not an 'on-call' service.
- DNA per cent: this includes all DNA and UTA for first and follow-up appointments as a percentage of all appointments.
- Validated clinical outcome measures used: identify at the bottom of the sheet the names of the validated outcome measures used.
- Community types: for each of these broadly defined types, enter the relevant data in each column. Some listed will not be relevant to all professional groups. It is anticipated that data will be provided for a wide range of specialties for each profession, but not necessarily every one.
- Other (please specify): if your community service is different from one in the list, please identify it and provide data; this may make it more difficult to benchmark, so only use when really necessary.

5. Community Services

Name of Your Professional Group:

	WTE Registered Staff									WTE Non-Registered Staff			Average no. new patients/ week per WTE	New patients last year	Total contacts last year	DNA %	1st : Follow-up ratio	Validated clinical outcome measures used? Yes/No
	Band 5	Band 6	Band 7	Band 8a	Band 8b	Band 8c	Band 8d	Band 9	Band 2	Band 3	Band 4	Band 5						
Adult Domiciliary																		
Intermediate care																		
Early Supported Discharge (stroke)																		
Neurology (excluding stroke)																		
Learning Disabilities																		
Paediatric Domiciliary																		
Other: HM Prisons																		
Other: Community Clinics																		
Total																		

Guidance:
Where there is no separation between Intermediate Care and Adult Domiciliary services, combine the two.

TABLE 5 Community services

The 7-days-a-week question – what staffing level?

If AHP services are essential to healthcare, and clearly they are, then it is reasonable to ask why aren't they universally provided for 7 days a week, every week of the year? Of course many AHP services or parts of them in specific clinical specialties are provided 7 days a week and there are also a range of 'on-call', stand-by and other out-of-hours and weekend services provided, but these arrangements are by no means universal.

AHP budgets are generally in the region of 90% staffing costs and it is often argued that it would not be possible to provide all AHP services across 7 days a week against the background of cash-strapped healthcare services. A further argument often advanced is that 7-days-a-week services could be provided without increased costs. However, it is clear that most things have a cost, in terms of finance or by loss of service during Monday to Friday if services are taken out to be spread across the whole 7 days. The 'no cost' to spreading the 5-days-a-week service across the 7-day week simply does not stand up. Decreasing service provision during the Monday to Friday period must have an adverse effect on care provision and the outcomes of services working to optimal clinical capacity during this period. If the service is not working to optimal capacity then this is a management issue which needs to be dealt with in its own right. The effect of moving some service capacity from 5 days per week to cover all 7 days of the week is clearly demonstrated by the illustration in Figure 5 below.

If, for example, optimal service provision for Monday to Friday is 20 units per day – total for the 5 days = 100 service units provision (20 × 5 days = 100); to use the same 100 units capacity for 7 days would result in 14.285 service units per day for each of the 7 days (100 units divided by 7 days =14.285 service units).

Monday	Tuesday	Wednesday	Thursday	Friday	Saturday	Sunday	Total staffing units WTE
20	20	20	20	20	X	X	100
14.285	14.285	14.285	14.285	14.285	14.285	14.285	100

FIGURE 5 Five to seven day workforce redeployment

This demonstrates that spreading the 100 WTE staffing units capacity over 7 days by taking units from Monday to Friday to cover Saturday and Sunday at a consistent level for the whole 7 days decreases Monday to Friday provision by 5.715 units on each of the 5 days from Monday to Friday; this is likely to have implications for the safety and effectiveness of the entire service.

This is a simplistic example as in many instances there is already a small level of service provision at the weekends. However, the principle is that if services are taken out of the 5-day period so that a 7-day service can be provided, then the cost is a decreased service during the 5 days through spreading the service more thinly. While flexibility is necessary in workforce deployment it is clear that extending the service from 5 to 7 days using the same total WTE staffing must have a clinical and quality cost; whichever way it is viewed, 7-days-a-week service provision has its cost. Some flexibility in workforce deployment is positive and helpful; however, to fund properly an increase in workforce to cover all 7 days is a necessary and more honest approach.

If the service was previously working optimally during the Monday to Friday period increases in the overall level of staffing will need to be put in place to maintain fully the Monday to Friday level of service. For the provision of a 7-days-a-week service, safe and effective staffing levels need to be set through the use of our methodology; that is, ascertaining all elements of the demand and then matching staffing to these requirements to balance the equation.

Care pathways in the context of staffing level determination

Over the last decade or two there has been increasing emphasis on the development of integrated care pathways in the NHS as a whole. An integrated care pathway may be defined as a plan of care that aims to promote organised and efficient multidisciplinary patient care based on the best available evidence. Care pathways can be complex interventions comprising a number of components provided by a range of clinical services and professions.[108] The question might arise about whether it is possible to use our methodology for determining staffing levels in situations where several AHPs and other disciplines are working in integrated interdisciplinary care pathway settings. In this event, the workload of individual professions within the multidisciplinary group can still be calculated, to work out the level of input required from any specific professional group; this is achieved by undertaking the calculations for each AHP group separately, then building the team to match identified workload.

Business cases

There are many possible ways of constructing business cases and the content will vary greatly in accordance with the specific requirements for the particular development proposal under consideration. In Appendix 3, we set out brief guidance notes on key elements for the structure and contents of a typical business case. As with so much around planning, development, option appraisal and the associated documentation, there is no single right or only one way of achieving the result, but hopefully this template (*see* Appendix 3) will serve as a useful aide-memoire. If the business case which you are developing is focused on staffing levels (for example, for a possible new service, service redesign or simply re-evaluating an existing service), detailed analysis, explanation and justification of all of the demand factors necessary for a safe, effective service which meets all the requirements and desired outcomes – and how these will be matched by the staffing supply proposed – are a crucial element of the document. In such cases the service requirement and the staffing required to match this demand element needs to be expanded, clear, precise and well argued. If the funding and other resources available for a new service are set out before the business case and option appraisal are commenced, and if this funding is not negotiable, then the service demand elements and the staffing to match the requirements will need to be modified realistically to ensure that the service can be provided safely and effectively within the resources available.

Conclusion

Our main objective for this chapter was to set out our methodology for determining safe and effective staffing levels, together with some of the tools and techniques we have developed to support application of the methodology. We have also included an appendix (Appendix 4) setting out a checklist for what we consider to be some of the most important data for AHP managers and leaders to have available, to support their work in staffing level determination and also in their wider management and leadership roles.

Our methodology is straightforward and logical and is firmly based on patient and service need, anticipated or agreed throughputs, activity volumes and desired outcomes, and the evidence-based real staff capacity and skill mix required to achieve this. Undoubtedly the methodology requires some work for collection of the necessary background data for each clinical service under review, new service plan, service redesign or new way of working.

In summary, we believe it is clear that the most logical and effective and efficient way to approach staffing level determination is to assess accurately the volume of work to be done at the standard required for safe and effective outcomes and set the staffing capacity to match this.

APPENDIX 1

HCPC professions

Professions	Numbers
Art therapists	3443
Biomedical scientists	21,777
Chiropodists/podiatrists	13,039
Clinical scientists	4868
Dietitians	8351
Hearing aid dispensers	1981
Occupational therapists	33,926
Operating dept practitioners	11,866
Orthoptists	1317
Paramedics	20,010
Physiotherapists	48,973
Practitioner psychologists	19,793
Prosthetists/orthotists	946
Radiographers	28,955
Social workers in England	88,474
Speech and language therapists	14,016

APPENDIX 2

Principles for computerised information systems for AHP services

Appendix 2 is intended as a brief guide to some of the key points for AHP managers and leaders to consider when embarking on development or implementation of computerised IM&T systems for their services. In discussion with AHP managers and leaders we have been surprised to find that many AHP services have inadequate or even no computerised support even this far into the 21st century, and therefore the information provided in this appendix is intended as a checklist of some of the important points to bear in mind when developing, renewing or implementing systems for the first time.

Many services have the information needed to undertake staffing levels work held in paper manual systems and will be able to supplement this with data from various computer systems within their organisations, but undoubtedly specific IM&T systems within AHP services will support this work.

Principles for computerised information systems for AHP services

1. **Information use**: all information collected should be for identified and agreed use. Computerised information systems should provide:
   - Information required for clinical, managerial and business purposes within AHP services locally.
   - Information required nationally or regionally.
   - Information required for the employing organisation.
   - Information required by commissioners and all other service purchasers and planners.

2. **Local ownership**: the computerised information system should be specific to the clinical and managerial/leadership needs of AHP services locally:

- Systems should be 'owned' by the AHP services using them locally, and part of the wider computer system within the organisation.
- Information contained within the system is 'owned' by the AHP services and the organisation.
- AHPs should be involved in the choice of appropriate information systems for their service.

3. **Computer hardware**: AHP services should have appropriate hardware to support their information systems, the hardware must:
   - Have the capacity to handle the quantity of data required at present and be capable of expansion to meet future needs.
   - Be capable of supporting a wide variety of applications.
   - Be capable of supporting a variety of input devices and terminals including adaptive equipment for sensory impaired users.
   - Be compatible with hardware used by other services and departments locally.
   - Be capable of supporting a variety of data collection modes such as data collection in 'real time', bar coding, personal digital assistants (PDAs), paper systems, retrospective input and so on.
   - Operate at the highest speed commensurate with the size of the information system locally.
   - Be capable of processing data in 'real time' and batch modes.

4. **Computer software**: computer software for AHP information systems should be appropriate to clinical and managerial/leadership practice; the software must:
   - Be specific to AHP requirements.
   - Be compatible with other programs used locally in order to facilitate interfacing/integration.
   - Enable archiving and retrieval of archived data.
   - Interface easily with other programs/applications such as Microsoft packages, programs for clinical purposes and other databases.
   - Interface with specialist software for sensory impaired users.
   - Be capable of updating in line with changing requirements.
   - Be designed to accommodate SNOMED, ICD and other coding systems.

5. **System security**: AHP systems must be secure so as to protect the confidentiality of patients, staff and others about whom data are held.
   - Data must be collected, processed and stored within the requirements of data protection legislation.
   - Entry to the AHP system must be governed by a system of passwords.
   - Staff must 'log off' computer equipment when not using it.
   - There must be full backup of data on a daily basis.

6. **Data collection**: all data collected by AHPs should – wherever possible – be a by-product of clinical practice:
   - All data collected by AHPs should be for identified and agreed use.
   - All patient intervention data items are collected once only if possible.
   - The data system must facilitate the collection, processing, analysis and reporting of locally agreed clinical and managerial information, as well as that required regionally and nationally; it must be possible to report on all parameters input to the system.
   - The system should facilitate the collection, processing, analysis and reporting of information about the use of AHP resources in patient-related activity and non-patient-related activity.
   - Data input to systems may be undertaken by clerical, clinical or managerial staff.

7. **Reporting**: the computer system must be capable of producing standard and ad hoc reports for AHP clinical, managerial/leadership, research and business purposes, as well as meeting the agreed requirements of others:
   - The system must be able to produce reports to support a wide range of business processes, such as service line reporting, costing and pricing, referral to treatment time (RTT) reporting, external contract requirements, commissioning, staff activity and throughput, capacity and demand.
   - The system must be able to produce reports to support a wide range of clinical processes, such as: audit, research requirements, clinical case loads, case mix, outcome measurement.
   - Computer reports must be available to AHP managers and clinicians as and when required.
   - Reports are easily accessible from the system in a variety of modes: tabular, bar charts, pie charts, spreadsheets, and so on.
   - The system should facilitate the design and generation of ad hoc reports as well as standard reports by AHP managers and clinicians as well as others within the organisation.

8. **Service agreements**: there must be service agreements with computer companies supplying the AHP system:
   - There must be service agreements for the computer software with agreed 'call-out' and support response times.
   - Agreements should include, for example, systems failure, maintenance, support, trouble shooting, further developments.
   - It is helpful if there is a user group attended by the software company that the AHP manager can participate in.

9. **Computer system documentation**: there must be full documentation for the software:
   - Comprehensive manual on the computerised information system software use.
   - User manuals.
   - Coding manuals.
   - Report templates.

10. **Staff training**: training at all levels on use of the system must be provided:
    - Training must be provided for clerical and reception staff.
    - Training must be provided for AHP staff.

APPENDIX 3

Key elements in a business case

Different organisations may have their own templates for business case submission; however, if there is no set format the following is a useful guide. Ensure essential information is included such as: name of the organisation, name of the service, author(s), contact details and date. Presentation is very important, as is the accuracy and relevance of the contents.

Elements in a business case – an example
- Contents list:
- Date:
- Name of division/department or service:
- Business case for:
- Business case Author(s):
- Divisional Clinical Director:

Executive summary
A brief overview of the business case, current situation, options, preferred option, financial details and recommendation(s).

Introduction and purpose of the business case
This includes an explanation of what the business case is about and why it has been prepared, what services(s) you are aiming to provide, for whom, where, when and why. Set out an outline of the business case content and mention the option appraisal, stating that the preferred option for the directorate is …

Description and analysis of reasons for the business case
Local context
Explain what services are currently available, what the issues are, why something new, different or extra is required, what the gaps are and what would be needed to improve services or resolve the problem. This might include, for example, delays in access to treatment, long waits, no service available, waiting

list information, service only available in other areas, information about relevant audits which have been undertaken, clinical governance issues, expertise available and so on.

Strategic context and headlines
Include a range of relevant information, for example:
- Fit with the organisation's strategy.
- High impact changes.
- Referral to treatment times (where applicable).
- National service frameworks.
- NICE recommendations (where applicable).
- Local and national guidelines.
- Targets set by the organisation, commissioners or nationally.
- Summary of the challenges and what the outcome is likely to be if the challenge is not addressed.

Options
For the Option appraisal, number and provide headings for each option. This could be set out in columns, for example:

Option 1
- Column 1 – Description of option – might be to do nothing.
- Column 2 – Advantages of option – brief list of advantages.
- Column 3 – Disadvantages of option – brief list of disadvantages.
- Column 4 – Total cost pa – revenue and capital.

Option 2
- Similar format, except that column 1 will describe a specific option.
- Columns 2, 3 and 4, as above.

Option 3
- Column 1 – Description of a further option.
- Columns 2, 3 and 4 as above.

Generally, the Options appraisal will include three or four options.

Ranking, preferred option and benefits
In this section rank the options in order of preference and provide an explanation of why a specific option is preferred, benefits and so on (benefits realisation).

Risk analysis
Outline the risks involved in implementation of each option and the risks involved in not implementing.

Impact on other divisions/directors within the organisation

Give an outline of whether the proposal impacts on other divisions, directorates or services within the organisation in terms of, for example:
- Staffing.
- Use of facilities and equipment.
- Timetabling.

APPENDIX 4

Suggested data checklist for AHP managers and leaders

We have found these data items to be essential to a variety of AHP management and leadership roles and tasks. This list is not exhaustive, but is intended as a checklist to ensure appropriate data are available at any time they are required. The list is not in priority order.

- WTE registered staff working in each part of the service, e.g. department, section, specialty, unit, etc.
- Total WTE registered staff within the whole service by profession.
- WTE assistant staff working in each area (non-HCPC Registered).
- Total WTE assistant staff.
- WTE administration and clerical staff working in each area.
- Total WTE administration and clerical staff in your service.
- Number of patients referred to the service(s) in the last financial year and the same for several previous years.
- Patient throughput in each clinical area, section, unit, etc. last financial year and for several previous years.
- Total number of patient throughput in the financial year and for several previous years.
- Number of patient face-to-face contacts in the last financial year and for several previous years (broken down into per month, per week, per day) by whole service, professions, and for clinical specialties, departments, units, etc.
- Average number of referrals (new patients) per year per WTE member of staff in each specialty, unit, department, etc.
- Average number of referrals per WTE by profession per week.
- Number of treatment slots available each week for new patients (out-patient services).
- Number of slots available each week for follow-up appointments.
- Work capacity available for in-patient and community services.
- Length of time for each out-patient new referral (new patient slot).

- Length of time for follow-up patient slot.
- Number of out-patient 'DNA' (did not attend includes unable to attend, i.e. all patients who were allocated an appointment and did not come) pa.
- Ratio of new patients to follow-ups.
- Waiting time in months, weeks, days (an average over the last year) and comparison with previous years.
- Activity levels, i.e. first and follow-up contact information by different staff grades/bands, AHP groups.
- Any activity data available on percentage time spent on patient-related activity and non-patient-related activity.
- Patient clinical data form – minimum data set:
  —Name of patient
  —NHS number
  —Permanent address
  —Date of birth
  —Occupation
  —Referred by
  —Any clinical follow-up appointments?
  —Hospital transport required (Y – N)
  —Telephone contact
  —GP
  —Consultant
  —Referral date
  —Therapy appointment date
  —Diagnostic code
  —Date of onset
  —X-ray reports
  —Medication
  —Home situation/support
  —Relevant medical history
  —Therapy reason for referral
  —Care group: NHS, private patient, overseas visitor
  —Therapy clinician code
  —Number of contacts in completed episode
  —Outcomes
  —Audit codes as appropriate
  —Discharge date
  —Discharge status
  —Home assessment visits
  —Appliances/equipment issued

APPENDIX 5

Numbers of Hospital Beds and Staff per 1000 population – examples of calculation

Calculating Beds to Population

Calculating number of beds per 1000 population
Divide number of beds in hospital by the number in the population served and multiply by 1000.

Example 1:
- 874 beds
- 361,000 population
- To find number of beds per person divide 874 by 361,000 = 0.0024 beds per person
- For beds per 1000 population multiply this figure by 1000.
- 874/361,000 = 0.0024 x 1000 = 2.4 beds per 1000 population

Example 2:
- 634 beds
- 253,000 population
- 634/253,000 = 0.0025 beds per person
- 0.0025 x 1000 = 2.5 beds per 1000 population

Calculating numbers of staff in a discipline per 1000 population

To work out how many staff in a given profession per 1000 population use the same methodology i.e. Divide number of staff by population and multiple by 1000

- 50 staff
- 300,000 population
- 50/300,000 = 0.00016 x 1000 = 0.16 staff per 1000 population

References

1. Francis R. *Report of the Mid Staffordshire NHS Foundation Trust Public Inquiry 1 January 2005–March 2009 Volume I. Chapter 23*. London: Department of Health; 2013. www.midstaffsinquiry.com/assets/docs/Inquiry_Report-Vol1.pdf
2. Williams JI. *Calculating Staffing Levels in Physiotherapy Services*. Rotherham: PAMPAS Publishing; 1991.
3. Williams JI. *No.1 Caseload, Casemix, Workload and Costing*. Doncaster Health Authority Physiotherapy Service; 1985.
4. Williams JI. *No.2 Monitoring Effectiveness in Physiotherapy Services*. UK: Doncaster Health Authority Physiotherapy Service; 1986.
5. Williams JI. *No.3 Measuring Efficiency in Physiotherapy Services*. UK: Doncaster Health Authority Physiotherapy Service; 1986.
6. Parliamentary Health Select Committee. *Third Report. After Francis: Making a Difference*. London: UK Parliament; 2013.
7. Department of Health. *Hard Truths; the Journey to Putting Patients First. The Government response to the mid Staffordshire NHS FT Public Inquiry*. London: HMSO; 2013. www.gov.uk/government/organisations/department-of-health
8. www.nice.org.uk/newsroom/news/NICEToProduceGuidanceSafeNHSStaffingLevels.jsp
9. Care Quality Commission. *Board Meeting 31 July 2013*; www.youtube.com/watch?v=4_CVKQCoZAs
10. Berwick D. *A Promise to Learn – a Commitment to Act. Improving the Safety of Patients in England*. London: National Advisory Group on the Safety of Patients in England; 2013. www.gov.uk/government/uploads/system/uploads/attachment_data/file/226703/Berwick_Report.pdf
11. Keogh B. *Review into the Quality of Care and Treatment Provided by 14 Hospital Trusts in England: Overview Report*; 2013. www.nhs.uk/NHSEngland/bruce-keogh-review/Documents/outcomes/keogh-review-final-report.pdf
12. Cavendish C. *The Cavendish Review: An Independent Review into Healthcare Assistants and Support Workers in the NHS and Social Care*; 2013. www.gov.uk/government/uploads/system/uploads/attachment_data/file/236212/Cavendish_Review.pdf
13. King's College London. *Safe Staffing Alliance Statement*; 2013. www.kcl.ac.uk/nursing/research/nnru/news/Alliance-Statement-May-2013.aspz
14. Research Services National Assembly for Wales. *Nurse Staffing Levels on Hospital Wards*. Cardiff: Research Services National Assembly For Wales; July 2013. www.assemblywales.org/RN13-012.pdf
15. National Assembly for Wales. *Plenary. RoP*. 12 March 2013. www.assemblywales.org/docs/rop_xml/130312_plenary_bilingual.xml
16a. National Assembly for Wales. *Plenary. RoP*. 17 April 2013. www.assemblywales.org/docs/rop_xml/130417_plenary_bilingual.xml
16b. National Assembly for Wales. www.assemblywales.org/bus-legislation/bill_ballots/bill-046.htm
17. Scottish Government. *Nurse Staffing Levels Available*; 2013. www.scotland.gov.uk/News/Releases/2012/11/staff261112
18. BBC. *Nurse leaders issue warning over staff numbers*. 12 May 2013. www.bbc.co.uk/news/health-22481151
19. Department of Health. *Compassion in Practice, Nursing, Midwifery and Care Staff, Our Vision and Strategy*; 2012. www.england.nhs.uk/wp-content/uploads/2012/12/compassion-in-practice.pdf

20. Cooper C. 'Jeremy Hunt urged to set NHS Safe Staffing Levels after Mid Staffs Scandal'. Independent.co.uk, 4 August 2013. www.independent.co.uk/life-style/health-and-families/health-news/jeremy-hunt-urged-to-set-nhs-safe-staffing-levels-after-mid-staffs-scandal-8747244.html
21. Keogh K. One in ten nurses fears a repeat of Mid Staffs where they work. *Nursing Standard.* 2013; **27**(37): 5.
22. Kay J. *The Case for Increased Nurse Staffing Levels.* HSJ.co.uk. 20 August 2013. www.hsj.co.uk/5059440.article
23. Royal College of Nursing. *Nurses condemn unsafe staffing levels.* 14 May 2013. www.rcn.org.uk/newsevents/news/article/uk/nurses_condemn_unsafe_staffing_levels
24. Moore A, Waters A. Getting ratios right, for the patients' sake. *Nursing Standard.* 2012; **26**(31): 16–19. http://nursingstandard.rcnpublishing.co.uk/campaigns/care-campaign/features/getting-ratios-right-for-the-patients-sake
25. Nursing Times. *Staffing levels – who's counting?* 31 July 2013. Nursingtimes.co.uk. www.nursingtimes.net/nursing-practice/healthcare-it/staffing-levels-whos-counting/5061867.article
26. The Guardian. 'Hospital Watchdog warns 17 have unsafe staffing levels'. Guardian.co.uk. 13 January 2013. www.theguardian.com/society/2013/jan/13/hospital-watchdog-17-unsafe-staffing/print
27. *Health Service Journal. Minimum safe staffing work yet to begin.* HSJ.co.uk. 23 August 2013. www.hsj.co.uk/news/exclusive-work-not-started-on-minimum-safe-staffing-levels/5062250.article
28. *Health Service Journal. Francis calls for rethink on minimum nurse staffing.* HSJ.co.uk. 6 August 2013. www.hsj.co.uk/news/francis-calls-for-rethink-on-minimum-nurse-staffing/5062029.article
29. *Health Service Journal.* www.hsj.co.uk/news/exclusive 20/08/201321
30. National Nursing Research Unit. *Registered Nurse Staffing Levels and Patient Outcomes.* London: King's College London; 2013.
31. Rafferty AM, Clarke SP, Coles J, et al. Outcomes of variation in hospital nurse staffing in English hospitals: cross-sectional analysis of survey data and discharge records. *Int J Nurs Stud.* 2007; **44**(2): 175–82.
32. Griffiths P, Ball J, Rafferty AM, et al. Nurse, care assistant and medical staffing: the relationship with mortality in English Acute Hospitals'. RCN Research Conference, March 2013.
33. Kane RL, Shamliyan TA, Mueller C, Duval S, Wilt TJ. The association of Registered Nurse staffing levels and patient outcomes: systematic review and meta-analysis. *Med Care.* 2007; **45**(12): 1195–1204. 10.10197/MLR.0b013e3181468ca3.
34. Needleman J, Buerhaus P, Pankratz VS, et al. Nurse staffing and inpatient hospital mortality. *N Engl J Med.* 2011; **364**(11): 1037–45.
35. Ball J, Murrells T, Rafferty AM, Griffiths P. *Care Left undone by Nurses in English National Health Service (NHS) Hospitals; the Association with Staffing Levels, Perceived Quality and Safety of Nursing Care.* BMJ Quality & Safety; 2013. http://qualitysafety.bmj.com/content/early/2013/07/08/bmjqs-2012-001767.full.pdf
36. Ball J, Pike G, Griffiths P, et al. *RN4CAST Nurse Survey in England, 2012.* King's College: London; 2012.
37. Royal College of Nursing. *RCN Policy Position: Mandatory Nurse Staffing Levels.* London: RCN; 2012. www.rcn.org.uk/__data/assets/pdf_file/0010/493282/03_12_Mandatory_nurse_staffing_levels_v2_FINAL.pdf
38. Griffiths P. *Care Left Undone.* University of Southampton; 2013.
39. Royal College of Nursing. *RCN Policy Position: evidence-based nurse staffing levels.* London: RCN; 2010. www.rcn.org.uk/frontlinefirst
40. Nursing Standard. Three-year review of staffing levels. *Nursing Standard.* 2013; **27**(46): 8.
41. Wales Professional Nurse Staffing Group. *Planning Nurse Staffing Levels on Acute Wards in Wales.* Cardiff: Wales Professional Nurse Staffing Group (undated).
42. Royal College of Nursing. Safe staffing for older people's wards: an RCN toolkit. www.rcn.org.uk/__data/assets/pdf_file/0009/479349/004301.pdf

43. Royal College of Nursing Policy Unit. *Setting Appropriate Ward Nursing Staffing Levels in Acute Trusts.* London: RCN; 2006.
44. Royal College of Physicians. *Setting Higher Standards: Consultant Physicians working with Patients,* Revised 5th edn. 2013. www.rcplondon.ac.uk/sites/default/files/consultant_physicians_revised_5th_ed_full_text_final.pdf
45. Royal College of Physicians. *Patient Safety Policy.* 2011. www.rcplondon.ac.uk/policy/improving-healthcare/patient-safety
46. Royal College of Physicians. *Commission in Improving Dignity in Care for Older People: Royal College of Physicians' Evidence.* London: RCP; 2011.
47. Royal College of Physicians. *RCP Comment on Berwick Report.* London: RCP; 2013. www.rcplondon.ac.uk/press-releases/rcp-comment-berwick-report
48. British Association of Art Therapists. Email to Robert Jones. 3 June 2013 (unpublished personal communication).
49. The British Dietetic Association. Email to Robert Jones. 3 June 2013 (unpublished personal communication).
50. College of Occupational Therapists. Email to Robert Jones. 13 August 2013 (unpublished personal communication).
51. Royal College of Speech and Language Therapists. *Calculating hours available to a FTE Speech and Language Therapist.* www.rcslt.org/members/publications/managers_resources/calculating_available_hours.pdf
52. Royal College of Physicians. *National Clinical Guideline for Stroke,* 4th edn; 2012. www.rcplondon.ac.uk/sites/default/files/national-clinical-guidelines-for-stroke-fourth-edition.pdf
53. Royal College of Physicians. *National Sentinel Stroke Audit 2010.* London: RCP; 2010. www.rcplondon.ac.uk/sites/default/files/national-sentinel-stroke-audit-2010-public-report-and-appendices_0.pdf
54. Skrypak M, Basu-Doyle M, Barron S. Acute care. Support for early stroke discharge. *Health Serv J.* 2012; **122**: 24–5.
55. British Society of Rehabilitation Medicine. *Rehabilitation Following Acquired Brain Injury: National Clinical Guidelines.* London: Royal College of Physicians; 2003.
56. The British Dietetic Association. *The Value of Nutrition and Dietetics for Stroke Survivors;* 2007. www.eoe.nhs.uk/downloadFile.php?doc_url=1341224771_LnGB_the_value_of_nutrition_and_dietetics_in_stroke_car.pdf
57. Scottish Intercollegiate Guidelines Network. *Management of Patients with Stroke: Rehabilitation, Prevention and Management of Complications, and Discharge Planning. A National Clinical Guideline;* 2010. www.sign.ac.uk/guidelines/fulltext/118/
58. Royal College of Speech and Language Therapists. *Communicating Quality 3: RCSLT's Guidance on Best Practice in Service Organisation and Provision.* London: RCSLT; 2006.
59. Royal College of Speech and Language Therapists. *RCLST Resource Manual for Commissioning and Planning Services for SLCN.* London: RCSLT; 2010.
60. Royal College of Speech and Language Therapists. *Quality Self-Evaluation Tool. (Q-SET)* London: RCSLT; 2006. www.rcslt.org/account/login?d=http%3A%2F%2Fwww.rcslt.org%2Fmembers%2Fprofessional_standards%2Fintro
61. Welsh Assembly Government. *Together Against Stroke.* Cardiff: Welsh Assembly Government; 2012.
62. National Cancer Action Team. *National Cancer Rehabilitation Workforce Mapping Exercise 2009: Comparative Report.* London: National Cancer Action Team; 2010.
63. Welsh Assembly Government. *National Standards for Head & Neck Cancer Services.* Cardiff: Welsh Assembly Government; 2005.
64. Welsh Assembly Government. *Designed to Improve Health and the Management of Chronic Conditions in Wales: An Integrated Model and Framework.* Cardiff: Welsh Assembly Government; 2007.

REFERENCES

65. British Society of Rehabilitation Medicine. *Rehabilitation Following Acquired Brain Injury: National Clinical Guidelines*. London: Royal College of Physicians; 2003.
66. British Psychological Society. *Briefing Paper 5: Commissioning Clinical Psychology Services for Older People, their Families and Other Carers*. London: BPS; 2006. www.bpsshop.org.uk/DCP-Briefing-Paper-No-5-January-2006-Commissioning-Clinical-Psychology-Services-for-older-people-their-families-and-other-carers-P754.aspx
67. British Psychological Society. *Occasional Paper no. 4. April 2002 Coronary Heart Disease National Service Framework: Cardiac Rehabilitation – Meeting the Information Needs*. London: BPS; 2002. www.cardiacrehabilitation.org.uk/nacr/docs/PHO_Article.pdf
68. British Association for Counselling and Psychotherapy. *Guidance For Best Practice – the Employment of Counsellors and Psychotherapists in the NHS*. UK: BACP; 2004. www.bacphealthcare.org.uk/members/guidance.php
69. Association Luxembourgeoise Kinésithérapeutes. Email to Robert Jones. 30 May 2013 (unpublished personal communication).
70. Norwegian Physiotherapist Association. Email to Robert Jones. 30 May 2013 (unpublished personal communication).
71. Irish Society of Chartered Physiotherapists. Email to Robert Jones. 7 June 2013 (unpublished personal communication).
72. German Federal Association for Physiotherapy. Email to Robert Jones. 28 June 2013 (unpublished personal communication).
73. Physiotherapy New Zealand. Emails to Robert Jones. 30 May 2013, 7 June 2013 (unpublished personal communication).
74. Dwyer, M. *Staffing Levels*. PT. Health Policy and Administration of the American Physical Therapy Association. 2012. http://hpaapta.wordpress.com/2012/06/26/staffing-levels/
75. Copeland J. *Survey Results Staffing Numbers 2008*. NZ: New Zealand Society of Physiotherapists Inc; 2008.
76. Royal Australian College of Physicians, Australian Faculty of Rehabilitation Medicine. *Standards for the Provision of Adult Rehabilitation Medicine Services in Public and Private Hospitals*. Aus: RACP; 2011.
77. Indian Health Service. *Planning, Evaluation & Research, RRM Category: AMBULATORY CLINICS, RRM Module: Physical Therapy*. (undated). www.ihs.gov/planningevaluation/index.cfm?module=rrm-ac-physical-therapy
78. Nursing Standard. Evidence shows staff. *Nursing Standard*. 2013; **27**(43): 20–2.
79. Association of District and Superintendent Chartered Physiotherapists. *Manpower: a Working Party Report*. London: ADSCP; 1980.
80. Jones R. *Management in Physiotherapy*. Oxford: Radcliffe Medical Press; 1991.
81. Curtis P, Rathwell T. *An Analysis of Physiotherapist's Work Activities*. Leeds: The Nuffield Institute, University of Leeds; 1987.
82. Wessex RHA Physiotherapy Working Group. *Report of the Working Group Set up to Examine Future Services and Manpower Requirements for the Physiotherapy Services*. Winchester: Wessex RHA; 1987.
83. Institute of Manpower Studies. *Understanding Physiotherapy Staffing Levels*. IMS Report No. 226. London: Association of Chartered Physiotherapists in Management; 1992.
84. ACPM, CSP Working Party. *Recommendations for Calculating Physiotherapy Staffing for GP Referred Musculoskeletal Outpatient Services*. UK: ACPM/CSP; 2002.
85. Beaumont K, Thornton J, Sleney H. *Physiotherapy: An Examination of Demand and Supply Issues*. London: Manpower Planning Advisory Group; 1989.
86. McKenna M, Maynard A, Wright K. *Is Rehabilitation Cost Effective?* York: Centre for Health Economics, University of York; 1992.

87. Oakley P, Practices Made Perfect Ltd. *Part 1 The Management Report. Providing Therapists' Expertise in the New NHS: Developing a Strategic Framework for Patient Care.* London: Department of Health; 1997.
88. Department of Health Statistics Division 3G. *NHS Physiotherapy Services Summary Information for 2003–04 England.* London: Department of Health; 2004.
89. British Geriatrics Society. 'Silver Book'; Quality Care for Older People with Urgent and Emergency Care Needs. 2012. www.bgs.org.uk/campaigns/silverb/silver_book_complete.pdf
90. Squires A, Hastings M. Physiotherapy with older people: calculating staffing need. *Physiotherapy.* 1997; **83**(2): 58–64.
91. Standing S, Eales H, Hurst A, et al. *Calculating Physiotherapy Staffing Levels within a Service for People with Learning Disability.* London: Association of Chartered Physiotherapists for People with Learning Disabilities; 2002.
92. PPIMS. *Nottingham Management Tool.* 2003. www.apcp.org.uk/APCPSpecialistGroups/PPIMS/NottinghamDemandManagementTool/tabid/221/ctl/Login/language/en-US/Default.aspx?returnurl=%2fAPCPSpecialistGroups%2fPPIMS%2fNottinghamDemandManagementTool%2ftabid%2f221%2flanguage%2fen-US%2fDefault.aspx
93. National AHP and HCS Critical Care Advisory Group. *Allied Health Professionals (AHP) and Healthcare Scientists (HCS) Critical Care Staffing Guidance.* UK: Department of Health; 2003.
94. AHPs, NHS Scotland. *AHP Capacity Calculator – User Guide.* Edinburgh: NHS Scotland; 2009. www.workforceplanning.scot.nhs.uk/media/14960/2.2%2014th%20may%202009%20kms%20ahp%20capacity%20calculator%20user%20guide.doc
95. The All Wales Physiotherapy Managers Committee. *Staffing Ratio Tool (Calculating Qualified Staffing Requirements for the Physiotherapy Profession in Wales).* Cardiff: The All Wales Physiotherapy Managers Committee; 2006.
96. Health and Social Care Information Centre (HSCIC). Email to Robert Jones. 5 July 2013 (unpublished personal communication).
97. Health Care Professions Council. Email to Robert Jones. Staffing Numbers in Physiotherapy Services. 12 September 2013 (unpublished personal communication).
98. NHS Benchmarking Network. *Acute Therapies Benchmarking Phase 3 Report.* London: NHS Benchmarking Network; 2013.
99. NHS Electronic Staff Record. www.electronicstaffrecord.nhs.uk
100. Ozcan S, Hornby P. *World Bank Health Project.* Ministry of Health, Ankara, Turkey and Centre for Health Planning and Management, Keele University, England; 2011. www.who.int/hrh/en/HRDJ_3_3_05.pdf
101. Shipp PJ. *Internal Report.* Jarkata: Planning Bureau, Ministry of Health; 1984.
102. Shipp PJ. *Workload Indicators of Staffing Need (WISN); a Manual for Implementation (Version 1).* Geneva: World Health Organization, 1989.
103. www.human-resources-health.com/content/10/1/2
104. Jones R, Jenkins F. *A Survey of NHS Physiotherapy Waiting Times, Workforce and Caseloads in the UK 2010–2011.* London: CSP; 2011.
105. Jones R, Jenkins F. *A Survey of NHS Waiting Times and Musculoskeletal Workload and Caseload in England.* Bath: JJ Consulting Healthcare Management Ltd; 2010.
106. Jones R, Jenkins F. *Key Tools and Techniques in Management and Leadership of the AHPs.* Milton Keynes: Radcliffe Publishing; 2011.
107. www.jjconsulting.org.uk
108. Jones R, Jenkins F. *Key Topics in Healthcare Management – Understanding the Big Picture.* Oxford: Radcliffe Publishing; 2008.

Index

7-days-a-week services 50, 68–9, **68**

ACPM (Association of Chartered Physiotherapists in Management) 35
activity analysis 4, 39, 50
activity sampling system 50, 52, 55–6
AfC (Agenda for Change) 39, 46, 53
After Francis report 4–5
Age UK 36
AGILE 36
AHP Capacity Calculator 37–8
AHP managers
    and activity analysis 50
    and benchmarking 56–8
    important data for 70, 79–80
    and information management 55–6
    and quality issues 45
AHPF (Allied Health Professions Federation) 23–4
AHPs (allied health professionals)
    activity data collection form **51**, 52–3, 55–6
    benchmarking tool 56–67
    documents and guidelines for 25–7, 38
    information services for 72–5
    need for sound data in 43
    professional bodies for 23–5
    staffing costs in 68–9
    staffing ratios of 30, 41
    staffing requirements for 46
    workforce planning for 40–1
    working week of 46–7
annual activity approach 3
assistant staff 79
Association of Chartered Physiotherapists for People with Learning Disabilities 36
Australia 11, 29–30, 41
AWPM (All Wales Physiotherapy Managers) 38

BDA (British Dietetic Association) 24
benchmarking 36, 49–50, 56–8
Berwick Report 8, 23

BPS (British Psychological Society) 26
Brearley, Sally 14
British Association of Clinical Psychologists 26
British Geriatrics Society 36
Buchan, Jim 15
business cases 4, 43, 69–70, 76–8

California 11
capacity, use of term 3
care assistants 18
Cavendish Review 8–9
CfWI (Centre for Workforce Intelligence) 22–4
CIP (cost improvement programmes) 2
clerical staff 60, 79
clinical data forms 80
clinical interest groups 25, 36–7
clinical staff, use of term 4
CNO (Chief Nursing Officer) 10
community services 57–8, 66–7, **67**, 79
complexity of cases 38
compliance regimes 19
Concise Guides for Stroke 26
COT (College of Occupational Therapists) 24
counsellors 26–7
CQC (Care Quality Commission) 5, 7, 9, 14, 17
CRES (cash releasing efficiency savings) 2
CSP (Chartered Society of Physiotherapy) 23, 33, 35–7

demand assessment 3
dementia services 26
dietitians 24, 58, 71
DNA (did not attend) 55, 64–7, 80
Drakeford, Mark 10

face-to-face patient contact 25, 46–8, 53
falls services 26
follow-ups 47–8, 80
Francis, Robert 5, 7–8, 13–15
Francis Report
    and staffing levels 1, 5, 7, 13

Welsh government response to 9–11

Germany 27–8
grade mix 3, 45
Griffith, Lesley 9–10
Griffiths, Peter 19

HCPC (Health and Care Professions Council)
    on AHP staffing 38
    professions covered by 46, 71
    registration with 44
Health Select Committee 4
healthcare assistants (HCAs) 4, 9, 18
hospital beds 81–2
HPA (Health Policy and Administration) 29

in-patient services 5, 57–8, 62–3, **63**, 66
Indian Health Service 30–1
information management 55–6, 72–5
Ireland 27

Keogh Report 8–9, 14

learning disabilities 36
LHBs (Local Health Boards) 9, 20
Luxembourg 27

Mandatory Nurse Staffing Levels 19
medical services 22, 62
Mid Staffordshire NHS Foundation Trust 1, 7–9, 13–14
multidisciplinary teams, staffing levels for 26

National Clinical Guideline for Stroke 25
National Nursing Research Unit 14, 17, 19
New Zealand 28–9, 48
NHS (National Health Service)
    AHPs in 4–5
    integrated care pathways in 69
    research on staffing levels in 1–3, 8
    work on staffing levels in 15, 17–18

INDEX

NHS Benchmarking Network 38–9
NHS Commissioning Board 11
NHS Electronic Staff Record 39
NICE (National Institute for Health and Care Excellence) 5–6
Northern Ireland 9, 20
Nottingham Demand Management Tool 36
Nuffield Institute for Health Service Studies 34, 56
nurse managers 18
nurse-to-patient ratios 19
nursing; *see also* registered nurses
   literature on staffing levels 31
   staffing levels in 9–11, 13, 15, 18–22
   support workers in 10

older people, staffing levels for care of 18, 23, 36
on-call services 62, 66, 68
option appraisal 4, 69–70, 76–7
organisations, general information on 58, **59**
OTs (occupational therapists) 24, 39
out-patient services **65**
   in benchmarking tool 64–5
   data on 80
   patient-related activity in **55**
   in physiotherapy 49
   provision of 28, 31
outcome measures 39, 62–4, 66

Paediatric Physiotherapists in Management Support Group 36
patient-related activity 48–50, 53, 56
patient safety
   and nurses 21
   and staffing levels 1, 7–8
physiotherapy
   children's needs for 36–7
   international staffing levels 27–31
   methodologies for staffing levels 33–5, 37–8
   in NHS Benchmarking Network 38–9
   workload data in 49
Planning Nurse Staffing Levels on Acute Wards in Wales 20
Poots, Edwin 20
Poulter, Dan 11
professional associations
   for AHPs 23–7
   for medical services 22–3
   in nursing 17–22
professional groups
   in benchmarking tool 57–60, **61**
   training for 53
   use of term 52
professional judgement 36–7
psychologists 25–6

RCN (Royal College of Nursing) 11, 14, 19–22
RCP (Royal College of Physicians) 22–3, 26
RCSLT (Royal College of Speech and Language Therapists) 24
rehabilitation medicine 30
RTT (referral to treatment time) 74

Safe Staffing for Older People's Wards 20
Scotland 9, 11, 20, 37
Sentinel audits 26
service capacity data 22
Setting Appropriate Ward Nurse Staffing Levels in NHS Acute Trusts 20–1
SIGN (Scottish Intercollegiate Guidelines Network) 26
Silver Book 36
social care organisations 24
SSA (Safe Staffing Alliance) 7–8, 11, 14, 18–19
staff activity analysis, *see* activity analysis
staff time, subdivision of **54**
staffing levels
   bodies setting 13
   calculating population ratio 82
   and care pathways 25, 69
   Jones/Jenkins methodology for 3–5, 43–5, 48–9, 70
   mandatory 10–11, 19
   media coverage of 13–15
   methodologies for determining 21, 31, 33–4, 36, 41–2
   professional organisations on 17–19
   and quality 2, 6
   research on 1–2, 36
   and workloads 49
staffing norms 5, 39–40
Staffing Ratio Tool 38
staffing ratios 27, 29, 31, 41
stroke services 25–6, 30, 46
support workers, Cavendish on 9

Turkey 39–40

United Kingdom, four countries of 9, 44
United States 29, 31
UTA (unable to attend) 55, 64, 66

Wales
   NHS services in 9–10
   physiotherapy staffing in 37–8
   workforce planning in 20
Ward sisters 18
WCPT (World Confederation of Physical Therapy) 27
Welsh Government 9–10, 20
White, Jean 10
Williams, Joyce 1, 24, 34–7, 40, 56
WISN (Workload Indicators of Staffing Need) 39–40
workforce planning
   flexibility in 5
   in nursing 20–2
   research on 40–1
working hours 40, 47, 52, 55
workload, data examples for 47–9
WTE (whole time equivalents) 1–2, 44